BDS & CBS India
Exam. Oriented Series

CONSERVATIVE DENTISTRY Inc. ENDODONTICS

(Questions & Answers)

Praveen Bansal

Foreword by
Dr. Ashok Dhoble

CBS

CBS PUBLISHERS & DISTRIBUTORS
NEW DELHI • BANGALORE (INDIA)

ISBN : 81-239-1459-8

First Edition : 2007

Reprint: 2008

Publishing Director : Vinod K. Jain

Published by :
Satish Kumar Jain for CBS Publishers & Distributors,
4596/1-A, 11 Darya Ganj, New Delhi - 110 002 (India)
E-mail: cbspubs@vsnl.com • Website: www.cbspd.com

Branch Office :
2975, 17th Cross, K.R. Road, Bansankari 2nd Stage, Bangalore-70
Fax : 080-26771680 • E-mail : cbsbng@vsnl.net

Composed by :
LineArt Graphics, Delhi-110091

Printed at :
India Binding House, Noida (UP).

Indian Dental Association

Dr. ASHOK DHOBLE
Hon. Secretary General
Bombay Mutual Terrace, 2nd Floor,
534, Sandhurst Bridge, Opera House,
Mumbai 400 007
Tel: 91-22-2364-3344/2363 6655
ashokdhoble@ida.org.in

Foreword

It gives me immense pleasure in presenting this series on Short Notes and Long Question Answer in Dentistry. The students of dental sciences face a difficult situation as they need to study their theory clubbed with clinicals and practicals. At the end of the year, although they may be good in their knowledge of theory and clinical skills, they still get tensed up due to lack of orientation towards university exam and the question paper pattern. This series has been designed specifically for this situation and I am sure it will go a long way helping the students in this direction.

Dr. Praveen Bansal is the brain behind this huge project and he took ideas and views from knowledgeable and experienced teachers, to write this series. The presentation style is catchy. I wish him all the best in this project as well as in his many more forthcoming projects.

Dr. ASHOK DHOBLE
Hon. Secretary General
Indian Dental Association, Head Office

Preface

BDS & CBS India Exam. Oriented Series is designed as pattern of long question answers, short question answers and clinical problems. The students are expected to know all the topic as well as specific information and last minute relevant details having clinical importance.

This series is structured to cover the essential aspects of BDS syllabus for quick reference in question answers format. I have tried my best to include almost all the topics presented in the syllabus by Dental Council of India in a simple language.

PRAVEEN BANSAL

Contents

Section–1

CONSERVATIVE DENTISTRY

Section–2

ENDODONTICS

Section–1

CONSERVATIVE DENTISTRY

1 Clinical Significance of Dental Anatomy and Physiology

S.Q.A.1 Different types of contact point & its importance in restorative dentistry ?

Ans. When teeth erupt to make proximal contact with previously erupted teeth, there is initially a contact point. The contact point becomes contact area because of wear of one proximal surface against another during physiologic tooth movements.

The proximal contact area is located in the incisal third of the approximating surfaces of the maxillary & mandibular central incisors. It is positioned slightly facial to the center of the proximal surface faciolingually. Procceding posteriorly from the incisor region through all the remaining teeth, the contact area is located near the incisal (or occlusal) & middle thirds or in the middle third. Because of these contacts being progressively lower cervically, larger incisal or occlusal embrasures result posteriorly.

Restorative procedures require maintenance of correct proximal contact relationships between teeth, which results in correct embrasures.

The properly formed & located proximal contacts promote normal healthy interdental papillae filling the interproximal spaces. Improper contacts can result in food impaction between the teeth, producing periodontal disease, carious lesions, & possible movement of the teeth. In addition, retention of food is objectionable by its physical presence & by the halitosis that results from food decomposition.

Proximal contacts & interdigitation of the teeth through occlusal contacts stabilizes & maintains the integrity of the dental arches.

S.Q.A.2 Dentin sensitivity ?

Ans. Sensitivity is encountered whenever odontoblasts and their processes are stimulated during operative procedures, even though the pain receptor mechanism appears to be within the dentinal tubules near the pulp. A variety of physical, thermal, chemical, bacterial & traumatic stimuli are transmitted through the dentinal tubules, though the precise mechanism of the transmissive elements of sensation has not been conclusively established.

Dentin hypersensitivity is a common clinical condition that is difficult to treat because the treatment outcome is not consistently successful.

Patients may complain of discomfort when teeth are subjected to temperature changes, osmotic gradients such as those caused by sweet or salty foods, or even tactile stimuli. The most accepted theory of pain transmission is the hydrodynamic theory, which accounts for pain transmission through small,rapid movements of fluid that occur within the dentinal tubules. Because many tubules contain mechanoreceptor nerve endings near the pulp, small fluid movements arising from cutting, drying, pressure changes, osmotic shifts, or changes in temperature account for majority of pain transmission.

The cervical area of teeth is the most common site of hypersensitivity. This cervical hypersensitivity may be caused not only by chemical erosion, but also by mechanical abrasion or even occlusal stresses.

Theories about the transmission of pain stimuli in dentin sensitivity suggest that pain is amplified when the dentinal tubules are open to the oral cavity. Therefore dentin hypersensitivity can be a major problem for periodontal patients who frequently have gingival recession and exposed root surfaces.

Clinicians have used many materials and techniques to treat this, including specific dentrifices, CO2 laser irradiation, dentin adhesives, antibacterial agents, aldehydes, resin suspensions, fluoride rinses, fluoride varnishes, calcium phosphate, potassium nitrate, & oxalates, among others.

2 Cariology

L.Q.A.1 Describe in detail the prophylactic treatment of dental caries

Ans. A caries prevention program is a complex process involving multiple interrelated factors. The primary goal of a caries prevention program should be to reduce the number of cariogenic bacteria.

Prevention should start with a consideration of the overall resistance of the patient to infection by the cariogenic bacteria. Although the General health of the patient,fluoride exposure history, & function of the immune system & salivary glands have a significant impact on the patient's caries risk, the patient may have little control over these factors. On the other hand, factors like diet, oral hygiene, use of microbial agents, & dental care are under patient's control.

Preventive treatment methods are designed to limit tooth demineralization caused by cariogenic bacteria, thereby preventing cavitated lesions.

These include:

- Limiting pathogen growth & metabolism
- Increasing the resistance of the tooth surface to demineralization.

Caries control methods are operative procedures used for both to stop the advance of individual lesions & to prevent the spread of pathogenic bacteria to other tooth surfaces & hence, are preventive procedures. These remove irreversibly damaged tooth structure & the associated pathogenic bacteria in the site.

Control procedures may also include pulpal therapy & restoration of damaged tooth surface to appropriate anatomic contours & function.

Management of dental caries & its consequences remains the dominant activity of dentists. The practitioner has to identify those patients with active carious lesions & those at a high risk of caries & institute appropriate preventive & treatment measures. Depending on the risk status of the patient the measures to be instituted is determined.

General health

The patient's general health has a significant impact on overall caries risk. The effectiveness of a patient's immunologic system is highly dependent on overall health status. Patient's undergoing radiation or chemotherapy treatment have significantly decreased immunocompetence and are at a risk for increased caries.

Medically compromised

Patients should be examined for changes in oral health. Early signs of increased risk includes increased plaque; puffy, bleeding gingival; dry mouth with red glossy mucosa & demineralization of the teeth. Decreased saliva is also vey common in acute and chronic systemic illness and hence increases plaque.

Fluoride exposure

In trace amounts increases the resistance of tooth structure to demineralization & is therefore a particularly important consideration for caries prevention. It produces spectacular decreases in the caries rate. The availability of fluoride to reduce caries risk is primarily achieved by fluoridated community water system & may also occur from fluoride in the diet, toothpastes, mouthrinses, & professional topical applications.

Immunization

The IgA immunoglobulins,(produced by the sensitized T & B cells in Peyer's patches along the intestinal walls,that migrate through the lymphatic system to bloodstream and finally are found in glandular tissues eg.salivary glands), are secreted in the saliva. These IgA antibodies are capable of agglutination of oral bacteria. This prevents adherence of the bacteria to the teeth and other oral structures, & they are more easily cleared from the mouth by swallowing.

This immunologic occurrence promotes the possibility of further vaccination against caries. However, it is known that the procedure is more effective against smooth surface than pit and fissure lesions.

Even if an anti caries vaccine were developed, concerns remain that may affect its widespread use.

First - Potential side effects;

Second - Cost of it &

Thirdly - Limitations imposed by governmental regulatory agencies.

Salivary function

Saliva is very important in prevention of caries. Lack of saliva greatly increases the incidence of caries. If patient is xerostomic, consultation with physician may be necessary to identify alternate treatments, if possible, with less salivary impact. Saliva stimulants (gums, paraffin waxes, or saliva substitutes) also may be prescribed for patients with impaired salivary functioning.

Antimicroblal agents

A variety of antimicrobial agents also are available to help prevent caries. Chlorhexidine is showing excellent results (mouthwashes, varnishes etc.).

The agent can also be applied professionally once a week for several weeks, monitoring the microbial counts to determine effectiveness. This may be used in combination with other preventive measures for high-risk patients.

Diet

Dietary sucrose has 2 important detrimental effects on plaque. First– provides stronger potential for MS colonization & second – mature plaque rapidly metabolizes sucrose to organic acids, hence causes profound and prolonged increase in plaque pH. Caries activity is most strongly stimulated by the frequency, rather than the quantity, of sucrose ingested.

Evidence of new caries activity in adolescent and adult patients indicates the need for dietary counselling. The goals of dietary counseling should be to identify the sources of sucrose in the diet and reduce the frequency of sucrose ingestion.

Oral hygiene

Daily removal of plaque by brushing, dental flossing and rinsing is the single best measure for preventing both caries and periodontal disease.

Pits and fissures are not accessible to tooth-brush bristles and so more susceptible to caries, obturation of these by sealants is a highly effective method.

A combination of oral hygiene and diet counseling is effective in children.

Rigid oral hygiene programs should be prescribed only to high-risk patients with evidence of active disease. Such cases need intensive oral hygiene training, dietary instruction & preventive dental treatment as necessary to control the progress of the disease. Frequent plaque removal, flossing,brushing & thorough rinsing after every meal is indicated.

Adults with low caries experience only require flossing, brushing & rinsing once a day.

Restorations

The status of a patient's existing restorations have an important bearing on the outcome of preventive measures and caries treatment. Old, corroded metallic restorations that are rough and hence plaque-retentive need smoothening & polishing or need to be replaced.

Restoration defects, such as overhangs, open proximal contacts & defective contours contribute to plaque formation and retention. Such defects need correction, usually by replacement of defective restoration.

Discoloration of enamel adjacent to a restoration, as a localized opalescent area, is suggestive of secondary caries.

The placement of restorations is preventive only in the sense of removing large numbers of cariogenic organisms & some of the sites in which they may be protected. The placement of restoration into a cavitated tooth in itself does not cure the carious process.

Preventive treatment is based on reducing the pathogen population size and increasing the resistance of the tooth to cariogenic attack. The most successful preventive treatment involves combination of all of the mentioned treatments, in a specific program designed for an individual that considers both caries and periodontal disease.

L.Q.A.2 Diagnosis of dental caries ?

Ans. The process of caries diagnosis involves risk assessment and the application of diagnostic criteria to determine the disease state. The primary objectives of caries diagnosis are to identify those lesions that require surgical (restorative) treatment, those that require nonsurgical treatment, and those persons who are at high risk for developing carious lesions.

Several factors must be considered while diagnosing. Some general factors like, patient history information and general clinical examination results, are helpful.

The emphasis in diagnosis must shift from detection of cavitations only to the detection of MS presence & predictions of caries progression.

Patient history

Factors include – age, gender, fluoride exposure, smoking habits, alcohol intake, medications, dietary habits, economic & educational status & general health.

Increased smoking, alcohol consumption, use of medications, and sucrose intake – high risk of caries development.

Children & elderly adults, patients with decreased fluoride exposure, lower economic status & lower educational attainment, poor general health – increases risk.

Clinical examination

Regarding inadequate salivary functioning, plaque accumulation, inflammation of soft tissues, poor oral hygiene, cavitated lesions & existing restorations help in determining the potential risk to caries development. More of these factors – greater the risk.

Assessing individual tooth surfaces for cavitation is crucial because restorative intervention becomes necessary. It is done primarily using visual assessment of discoloration, translucency or opacity. Injudicious use of sharp dental explorers on noncavitated, subsurface lesions could cause a cavitation.

Nutritional analyses

Frequent exposure to sucrose increases the likelihood of plaque development by the more cariogenic MS organisms.; these have been related to caries activity.

Salivary analyses

Provides information about appropriateness of secretion rates and buffering capacity as well as numbers of both MS & lactobacilli.

Radiographic assessment

Helps diagnosing carious lesions, the minimal depth of a detectable lesion on a radiograph is 500 ml. New techniques that may become available and useful include digital radiography, quantitative light-induced fluorescence, electrical conductivity, and ultrasonography.

Early detection of incipient caries, limitation of caries activity before significant tooth destruction has occurred, & identification of high-risk patients are primary goals of an effective diagnosis & treatment program.

Various diagnostic methods are available to detect caries activity at early stages.

These include:

- Identification of subsurface demineralization (inspection, radiographic, & dye uptake methods);
- Bacterial testing;
- Assessment of environmental conditions such as pH, salivary flow, & salivary buffering.

If failure to detect caries in its earliest stage occurs, caries is diagnosed by presence of cavitation of the tooth surface. The surface is examined visually & tactilely. Visual evidence includes cavitation, surface roughness, opacification & discoloration. Tactile evidence includes roughness & softness of the tooth surface. Roughness & softening have been determined by judicious probing of the suspected areas with explorer.

A single test for caries diagnosis usually cannot be used alone because such tests may not be sufficient for accurate caries diagnosis. Multiple criteria must be used and the diagnostic criteria should be adjusted according to the patient's overall risks (age,gender, fluoride exposure history,general health,& ability to maintain good oral hygiene).

3

Dental Materials

L.Q.A.1 Write the composition of glass ionomer cement ?

Ans. Glass Incomer cements are adhesive tooth colored anticariogenic restorative materials which were originally used for restorations of eroded areas.

This cement requires minimal cavity preparation as its bonds adhesively to tooth structure. Its named GIC because, the powder is glass & the setting reaction & adhesive bonding to tooth structure is due to ionic bond.

Classified as

Types I - For luting

Types II - For restorations

Types III - Liner & bases.

Also;

Types IV - Fissure sealants

Type V - Orthodontic cements

Type VI - Core build – up.

Can be included.

Composition - Powder / liquid in bottles:

Alumino silicate glass

It is similar to that of silicate, but has a higher alumina – silica ratio. This increases its reactivity with liquid.

Silica (SiO_2)	-	41.9
Alumina (Al_2O_3)	-	28.6
Aluminium fluoride (AlF_3)	-	1.6
Calcium fluoride (CaF_2)	-	15.7
Sodium flouside (NaF)	-	9.3
Aluminum phosphate ($ALPO_4$)	-	3.8

The fluoride component acts as a "Ceramic flux' lanthanum, strontium barium or zinc oxide additions provide rationality

Liquid

Earlier liquid was a 50 % aqueous solution of polyacrylic acid It was very viscous & had a tendency to gel.

- Polyacrylic acid
- Tartaric acids
- Water.
- Co polymerizing with iticonic, maleic acid etc. Tends to increase reactivity of the liquid decrease viscosity & reduce tendency for gelation.
- Tartaric acid improves the handling characteristics, increases working time & shortens setting time.
- Water is the medium of reaction & it hydrates the reaction products.

L.Q.A.2 What are polyacrylate cements? Write about extended uses of glass ionomer cement ?

Ans.

Polyacrylate cement

Cements that contain an aqueous solution of polyacrylic acid are termed as polyacrylate cement i.e. G.I.C.

Extended uses of GIC

- Originally, an esthetic restoration of anterior teeth & recommended for class III & V.
- As luting agents

- Restorative materials for conservative class-I & II cavities.
- Core build ups
- Pit & fissure sealants

Metal modified GIC: GIC have been modified by nclusion of metal filler particles to improve strength, fracture toughness & resistance to wear. Two methods have been employed:

Silver alloy admixed

Spherical amalgam powder mixed with type-II GIC (MIRACLE MIX)

Cermet

Silver particles are bonded to glass porticles. This is done by sintering of a mixture of the 2 powder at a high temperature (ketac silver)

Resin-modified GIC

Some polymerizing functional groups have been added to impart additional curing processes that can overcome the drawbacks of conventional GIC like moisture sensitivity & low early strength & allows the bulk of the material to mature through the acid-base reaction. Both chemical-curing & light-curing products are available.

L.Q.A.3 Adhesive restorations

Ans.

I. GLASS IONOMER CEMENT

Aluminium fluoride (AlF_3)	-	1.6
Calcium fluoride (CaF_2)	-	15.7
Sodium flouside (NaF)	-	9.3
Aluminum phosphate ($ALPO_4$)	-	3.8

- Glass Ionomer cements are adhesive tooth colored anticariogenic restorative materials which were originally used for restorations of eroded areas.
- This cement requires minimal cavity preparation as its bonds adhesively to tooth structure. Its named GIC because, the powder is glass & the setting reaction & adhesive bonding to tooth structure is due to ionic bond.

Classified as

Types I - For luting

Types II - For restorations

Types III - Liners & bases.

Also;

Types IV - fissure sealants

Type V - Orthodontic cements

Type VI - Core build – up.

Can be included.

Composition - Powder / liquid in bottles:

Alumino silicate glass

It is similar to that of silicate, but has a higher alumina – silica ratio. This increases its reactivity with liquid.

Silica (SiO_2) - 41.9

Alumina (Al_2O_3) - 28.6

The fluoride component acts as a "Ceramic flux' lanthanum, strontium barium or zinc oxide additions provide rationality

Liquid

Earlier liquid was a 50 % aqueous solution of polyacrylic acid. It was very viscous & had a tendency to gel.

- Polyacrylic acid
- Tartaric acids
- Water.

Uses

- Anterior esthetic restorative material for class III cavities
- For eroded areas & class V restorations
- As a luting agent
- As liners & bases
- For core build up
- To a limited extent as pit & fissure sealants

II. POLYCARBOXYLATE CEMENT

This was the first cement system developed with potential for adhesion to tooth structure.

Uses

- Primarily for luting permanent restorations.
- As bases & liners
- Used in orthodontics for cementation of bonds.
- Also used as rool canal fillings in endodontics

Available as

- Powder & liquid in bottles
- Water settable cements
- As precapsulated powder / liquid system
- Commercial names – Poly F, Durelon, Carboco.

Composition

Zinc oxide	-	Basic ingredient
Magnesium oxide	-	Principle modifier & also-
	-	aids in sitering
Oxides of bismuth & aluminium	-	Small amounts.
Stannous fluoride	-	Increases strength modifies setting time & imparts anti-cariogenic properties.

Liquid

- Aqueous solution of poylacrylic acid or
- Copolymer of acrylic acid with other unsaturated carboxylic acids, i.e iticonic maleic or tricarballylic acid.

Water settable cements

The polyacid is freeze dried & added to the cement powder. Water is used as the liquid when the powder is mixed with water, the polyacrylic acid goes into the solution & the reaction proceed as for the conventional cements.

Mixing time: 30 – 40 secs.

L.Q.A.4 Describe the composition, manipulation, resulting reactions and properties of silicate cements ?

Ans. Composition

Powder	Liquid
Silica (SiO_2) - 40%	Phosphoric acid - 92%
Alumina (Al_2O_3) - 30 %	Aluminium phosphate - 2 %
Sodium fluoride (NaF) - 19%	Cryolite (Na3 ALF6)
Zinc phosphate - 6%	Calcium phasphate or
$Ca(H_2PO_4)_2H_2O$ or -	
Magnesium phosphate	Lime (CaO)
Water - 40 %	

Manipulation

The liquid is dispensed just prior to mixing (other wise water evaporates & change the acid – water balance)

Powder / liquid ratio: 1.6 gm/ 4 ml.

Spatula used: Agate, plastic or cobalt - chromium spatula.

Steal spatulas are contraindicated as they get abraded by the silicate powder leading to discoloration of the mix.

Mixing time: One minute.

Resulting reactions: the ingredients of the cement powder are fused appox. 1400°C to form glass. The fluoride lowers the fusing temperature of the glass. The silicate glass powder is an acid-soluble glass. The liquid is an aqueous solution of phosphoric acid with buffer salts. When the powder & liquid are mixed, the surface of powder particles is attacked by the acid, releasing Ca2+, Al3+, & F- ions. The metal ions precipitate as phosphates that form the cement matrix with inclusions of fluoride salts. The chemistry of this material is virtually similar to GIC. The primary difference is that of the acid component of the liquid.

Properties

Physical properties

- Relatively strong in compression but weak in tension.
- Anticariogenic.
- Comparatively hard cement – 70 KHN.
- Gross leakage often occurs at the margins of silicate restoration.

Biologic properties

- pH is less than 3 at the time of insertion into cavity, & remains below 7 even after a month.
- Severe pulpal irritant, needs greater need for pulp protection.
- ***Dissolve and disintegrate in oral fluids:*** Relevance in anterior restoration: is an aesthetic material & hence used for anterior teeth. It is a fluoride containing cement, which eliminates sensitive bacterial populations. It has anticariogenic properties & a mechanism well defined – physiochemical mechanism & biologic mechanism of caries inhibition.

  Thus, it has been recognized that the incidence of caries is markedly less adjacent to the silicate restoration than that associated with all other filling materials. Also, the incidence of proximal surface adjacent to silicate is less than that of proximal surfaces adjacent to amalgam restorations.

L.Q.A.5 What are the reasons for placing a temporary restoration? List the materials used for temporary restoration? Write about one of the commonly used temporary restoration?

Ans. Between the time the tooth is prepared & the cast metal restoration delivered, it is important that the patient be comfortable & the tooth be protected & stabilized with an adequate temporary restoration. Temporaries can be fabricated intraorally directly on the prepared teeth-direct technique or outside of the mouth using a postoperative cast of the prepared teeth.

Materials used

1. Zinc-oxide eugenol cement.
2. Resin.

Zinc - Oxide eugenol cement

Cements of low strength and also are the least irritating of all dental cements & are known to have an abundant (sedative) effect on exposed dentin.

Classification

ADA Sq. NO 30: 4 types:

Types I ZOE - For temporary cementation

Types II ZOE - Permonent cementation

Types III ZOE - Tempory filling & thermal insulation

Types IV ZOE - Cavity liners.

Available as

- Powder & liquid
- Two paste system

Composition

Powder:

Zinc oxide	-	69% - principal ingredient
White resin	-	29.3%- To reduce brittleness of set cement
Zinc stearate - 1%	-	Accelerator plasticizer
Zinc acetate	-	0.7 % - Accelerator, improves strength
Magnesium oxide		

Liquid:

Eugenol	-	85% - Reacts with zinc oxide
Olive oil	-	15% - Plasticizer

Setting reaction is similar to ZOE paste

$Zn + H_2O \rightarrow Zn\ (OH)_2$

$Zn\ (HO)_2 + 2\ HE\ \ Zn\ E_2 + 2H_2O$

Base $\longrightarrow$ Acid Salt

(Zinc hydroxide) (Eugenol) (Zinc eugenolate)

The chelate formed is an amorphous gel that tends to crystallize imparting strength to the set mass.

Structure of set cement: Particles of ZO embedded in a matrix of zinc eugenolate.

Setting time: 4-10 mins. Set quickly in mouth due to moisture & heat.

Manipulation

Powder - liquid system: Ratio: 4: 1 to 6: 1 by wt.

- Bottles are gently shaken
- Measured guantity of both dispensed on or cool glass slab.
- Bulk of powder incorporated into liquid & saptulated thoroughly in a circular motion with a stiff bladed S.S. spatula.
- Smaller increments are than added until mix is complete.
- Oil of orange is used to clean eugenol cement from instruments.

Two paste system: Equal lengths of each paste are dispersed & mixed until a uniform color is observed.

L.Q.A.6 High copper amalgam / alloys

Ans. Contains more than 6% wt copper; these are preferred because of their improved mechanical properties, resistance to corrosion & better marginal integrity.

This is because the weakest γ–2 phase is eliminated here.

Types

- Admixed alloy powder
- Single composition alloy powder.

Admixed alloy powder

- Made by mixing 1 part silver – copper eutectic alloy (high copper spherical particles) with 2 parts silver tin alloy (low copper - lathe cut)
- These are stronger materials.

Composition

Silver - 60%

Tin - 17 %

Copper - 13 %

Zinc - 1 %

Setting reaction

- Silver enters mercury from the sliver copper eutectic alloy particles. And silver & tin both enter mercury from silver tin alloy.
- The mercury dissolved in silver-tin particles react like low copper alloys & form γ_1 & γ_2 phases with some unreacted silver-tin particles.
- Shortly the newly formed γ_2 phase will react with silver – copper forming eta or (n) phase.
- Some will also form around sliver-copper particles.

Reaction

Ag_3Sn + AgCu + Hg → Ag_2Hg_3 + Sn_3Hg + Ag_3Sn + Ag-Cu eutectic
(γ) (eutectic) (γ_1) (γ_2) (γ) unreacted & later,

Sn_6Hg + Ag – Cu → Cu_6Sn_5 + Ag_2Hg_3
(g_2) (eutectic) (η) (g_1)

Hence γ2 gets eliminated & is replaced by n phase.

Microstructure of set amalgam

Cu_6Sn_5 is present as a 'Halo' surrounding the Ag-Cu particles. Final set material consists of:

Core

- Unreacted Ag_3 Sn (γ phase) &
- Unreacted Ag – Cu, Surrounded by a halo of Cu_6Sn_5 (η)
- Matrix -γ_1 (Ag_2Hg_3)

Admixed high-copper

Advantages

- Longer working time

- Less dimensional change
- Displacement of matrix

Disadvantages

- Slower set
- High residual mercury
- Higher creep
- Less early strength
- Harder to finish

Spherical high-copper

Advantages

- Faster set
- Lower residual mercury
- Lower creep during condensation
- Faster finishing
- Higher early strength
- Low condensation pressure

Disadvantages

- Less working time
- Greater dimensional change
- Failure to displace malrix during condensation.

L.Q.A.7 Describe briefly the polishing procedure for amalgam ?

Ans. Most amalgams don't require finishing and polishing after the initial carving and burnishing. However, these procedures are occasionally necessary to:

- Complete the carving;
- Refine the anatomy, contours, & marginal integrity;
- Enhance the surface texture of the restoration.

Additional finishing & polishing procedures for amalgam restorations are not attempted within 24 hours of insertion, because crystallization is not complete.

An amalgam restoration is less prone to tarnish and corrosion if a smooth, homogenous surface is achieved.

Polishing of high-copper amalgams is less important than it is for low-copper amalgams, because high-copper amalgams are less susceptible to tarnish and marginal breakdown.

Finishing and carving reduces the initial roughness of a carved restoration. After polishing is completed, the tip of an explorer should pass from the tooth surface to the restoration surface without jumping or catching.

Initiate a polishing procedure by using a coarse, rubber abrasive point at low speed & air-water spray to produce an amalgam surface with a smooth satiny appearance.

Low speed is important for 2 reasons:

- The danger of the abrasive point disintegrating at high speeds.
- The danger of elevating the temperature of the restoration & the tooth.

An excessive temperature rise i.e. above 140°F can cause irreparable damage to the pulp or restoration or both. When overheated, the surface of the amalgam will appear cloudy even though it may have high polish. This cloudy appearance indicates the mercury has been brought to the surface, which results in corrosion of the amalgam & loss of strength.

After polishing with the coarse, abrasive rubber point, there should be no deep scratches on the amalgam surface, only the moderately polished surface left by the rubber point. In addition, the contour from tooth to restoration should be continuous when tested by the explorer tip.

After the area is washed free of abrasive particles, a high polish may be imparted to the restoration with a series of medium- & fine- grit abrasive points (at low speed). If a high luster does not appear within a few seconds, the restoration requires additional polishing with the more abrasive points. Using coarse-, medium-, fine-grit abrasive points in sequence will produce an amalgam surface with a brilliant luster. As an alternative to rubber abrasive points, final polishing may be accomplished using a rubber cup with a flour of pumice followed by a high-luster agent, such as precipitated chalk.

Polishing of older, existing restorations is infrequently indicated, only finishing may be indicated.

L.Q.A.8 Describe the causes of failure of amalgam restorations

Ans. Atleast 11 distinct conditions may be encountered when amalgam restorations are evaluated regarding its failures:

Amalgam 'blues'

Are discolored areas seen through the enamel. This bluish hue results either from the leaching of corrosion products of amalgam into the dentinal tubules or from the color of underlying amalgam as seen through translucent enamel. The latter occurs when the enamel has no dentin support, eg. Undermined cusps, marginal ridges & regions adjacent to proximal margins. Replacement may be considered for elective improvement of esthetics or for areas under heavy functional stress that may require a cusp capping restoration to prevent possible tooth fracture.

Proximal overhangs

Can be diagnosed visually, tactilely & radiographically. An explorer is moved back and forth across the amalgam-tooth junction, if it stops & then moves outwardly onto the amalgam, an overhang is present. Can also be confirmed by the catching or tearing of dental floss. Such overhangs can be a plaque trap, provide an obstacle to good oral hygiene, & result in inflammation of the adjacent soft tissue. Needs correction & indicates replacement of the defective restoration.

Marginal gap or ditching

Is the deterioration of the amalgam-tooth interface as a result of wear, fracture, or improper tooth preparation. Can be diagnosed visually or by explorer dropping into an opening as it crosses the margin. If the ditch is too deep to be cleaned or jeopardizes the integrity of the remaining restoration or tooth structure, the restoration needs replacement. In addition, secondary caries is frequently found around marginal gaps near the gingival wall & thus needs replacements.

Voids

Also occur at the margins of amalgam restorations. If the void is at least 0.3mm deep & is located in the gingival third of the tooth crown, then the restoration is judged as defective & should repaired or replaced. Accessible small voids in other marginal areas where the enamel is thicker may be corrected by recontouring or repairing with a small restoration.

Fracture line

A careful clinical examination will detect any fracture line across the occlusal portion of an amalgam restoration. A line that occurs in the isthmus region generally indicates fractured amalgam & thus a defective restoration that needs replacing.

Lines indicating the interface between abutted restorations

A manifestation of two abutted restorations, interface line, may be mistaken for fracture line. If other aspects of the abutted restorations are satisfactory, replacement is not needed.

Improper anatomic contours

Restorations that impinge on the soft tissue, have inadequate embrasure form or proximal contact, or prevent the use of dental floss should be classified as defective, indicating recontouring or replacement.

Marginal ridge incompatibility

The marginal ridge portion of amalgam restoration should be compatible with the adjacent marginal ridge. Both ridges should be at approximately the same level & display correct occlusal embrasure form for passage of food to the facial & lingual surfaces & for proper proximal contact area. If the marginal ridges are not compatible & are associated with poor tissue health, food impaction, or the inability of the patient to floss, the restoration is defective & should be recontoured or replaced.

Improper proximal contacts

Proximal area should touch the adjacent tooth at the proper contact level & with correct embrasure form. This is evaluated with dental floss & / or visually by trial angulations of a mouth mirror to reflect light & actually see if there is a space at the contact. if the contact is open & is associated with poor interproximal tissue health & / or food impaction, the restoration should be classified as defective & replaced as it is very annoying to the patient.

Recurrent caries – at the marginal area is detected visually, tactilely, or radiographically & is indication for repair or replacement.

Improper occlusal contacts: May cause improper, deleterious occlusal functioning & / or undesirable tooth movement. Needs correction or replacement.

L.Q.A.9 What is the composition of dental porcelain? Describe it.

Ans. Dental ceramics are the most suitable tooth suitable tooth colored restorative materials used to make denture teeth, single unit crowns, FPD's & labial veneers.

Most durable esthetic material, impervious to oral fluids & biologically compatible and chemically indestructible in most environment.

Composition

Feldspar	60 – 80 %	Basic glass former
Kaolin	3 - 5 %	Binder
Quartz	15 – 25 %	Filler
Aluumina	8 – 20 %	Glass former
Boric oxide	2 - 7 %	Glass former & flux
Oxides of na,	9– 15 %	Fluxes -K & Ca
Metallic pigments less than	1%	Colour matching.

Feldspar

Naturally occurring mineral & is a double silicate of potassium and Aluminium $K_{20} . Al_2O_3 . 6SiO_2$

- Acts as a flux matrix & surface glaze.
- When mixed with metal oxides & fired at high temperatures it can form a glass phase that able to soften & flow slightly. Hence porcelain powder particles coalesce together (sintering)
- It's the basic glass former. during firing, feldspar fuses & acts as a matrix & binds silica & kaolin.

Two important properties

- When fused at high temperature it retains its form without rounding.
- Between 1150° & 1530° it undergoes incongruent melting & forms crystals of leucite in a liquid glass.
- Leucite is a potassium aluminium silicate mineral with large co-efficient of TE.
- Incongruent melting is a process by which one material melts to form a liquid phus a different crystalline material.

Kaolin: Is a white lay like materials.

- Is a hydrated aluminum silicate
- Acts as a binder, gives opacity to mass.
- (substitutes - sugar or starch)

Silica: Is obtained by grinding pure quartz. Silica acts as a refractory skeleton & provides strength & hardness during fusing.

Aluminuim oxide: Replaces silica in glass matrix. Gives strength & opacity to the porcelain. Alters softening point & increases the viscosity.

Fluxes & glass modifires: These lower the fusion temperature & increase the flow of porcelain during firing. Can absorb or remove impurities.

If high flux concentration:

1. Reduces chemical durabilty of glass.
2. May cause glass to crystallize or devitrify

Coloring frits: There are produced by fusing various metallic oxides with fine glass & feldspar & then grinding to powder.

Added for various shades to match natural tooth color

Other Additions: Zirconium, titanium & tin oxide for color.

Manipulation

The porcelain powder is mixed with the liquid to form a plastic mass which is condensed to form the porcelain restoration.

Then it is fired in the furnace for sintering. When fired, the mass shrinks & flows, so the built up mass has to be supported on a matrix.

The matrix should have a higher fusion temperature than the porcelains.

Matrix

- Platinum foil of 0.001" is adapted on the die to form a wrinkle free matrix.
- Metal coping of suitable design & alloy.

The matrix supports the unfired porcelain. Before condensing, the matrix is degassed in the furnace to remove the gaseous impurities & anneal the platinum foil.

Building up porcelain

A plastic mass is prepared of porcelain powders mixed with liquid, with a brush the plastic mass is applied over the matrix.

It is built up to the shape of a crown. It is built up in a series of layers of core, dentine & enamel.

Condensation

The process of packing the powder particles together & removing excess water is known as condensation.

Purpose: Proper condensation packs the particles together, this helps minimize the porosity & reduce the firing shrinkage. & gives dense packing. Also helps to remove the excess water.

Technique

Vibration: Mild vibration by tapping or running a serrated instrument on the forceps holding the metal frame helps to pack the articles together & bring out the excess water. An ultrasonic vibrator is also available.

Spatulation: A small spatula is used to apply & smoothen the wet porcelain. This brings out excess water.

Dry powder: Is placed on the side apposite a wet increment. The water moves towards the dry powder pulling the wet particles together.

Ultrasonic: Mild vibration electrically.

Gravitational.

Whipping.

Firing

The process of sintering & fusing the particles of the condensed mass is known as firing.

The powder particles flow & fuse together; making. restoration dense & strong.

Firing is done in a porcelain furnace. After condensation, the compacted mass supported by the matrix should be placed. On a fire clay tray & inserted into the muffle of the ceramic or porcelain furnace.

The porcelain should novae be alloyed to come directly in contact with the walls & floor of the muffle.

The condensed mass is gradually heated by first placing it in from of the muffle of preheated furnace & later inserting into the furnace.

The entire program of preheating, firing subjecting to vacuum subjected to increased pressure. holding & cooling is known as FIRING CYCLE.

The firing cycles vary depending on stage-opaque firing, dentin firing, glaze firing etc. the temperature is lowered gradually for each subsequent firing cycle.

During firing, there is partial fusion of the particles at their point of contact. As temperatures is raised the fused glass gradually flows to fill up air spaces.

As the fused mass is viscous all the air cant escape & some get trapped giving rise to voids or porosity. Vacuum offset firing is done to reduce porosity in porcelain.

STAGES - Called bisque / biscuit stage:

Low bisque stage: Material becomes rigid & is very orous; very little shrinkage; particles lack cohesion & don't have translucency & glaze.

Medium bisque stage: Complete cohesion of powder particles. Its still porous, lacks translucency & high glaze There is definite shrinkage.

High bisque stage: Shrinkage is complete & mass exhibits smooth surface. Slight porosity may be seen. Body doesn't appear to be glazed.

At any stage, work can be removed, cooled & additions can be made.

Cooling: Slowly & uniformly done.

- It shrinkage not uniform, causes cracking & loss of strength.
- During cooling subsurface submicroscopic surface cracks occurs

L.Q.A.10 Finishing and polishing of composite restoration

Ans.

Finishing

Good technique & experience in inserting composite significantly reduce the amount of finishing required.

Slight excess of material present is removed with coarse diamond instruments, but generally not recommended for finishing because of the high risk of damaging contiguous tooth structure.

Steps

- Care to be taken with use of rotary instruments to not adversely affect adjacent tooth structure or teeth.
- A proper matrix with appropriate axial and line angle contours.
- Embrasures to be created to match the adjacent tooth embrasure form.
- No use of rotary instruments that leave roughened surfaces.
- A properly shaped contouring instrument for the area being contoured.
- The outline form to be prepared.
- The restoration to be viewed from all angles as it is contoured.

Effectiveness of restoration finishing & polishing procedures depends on careful use of successively finer abrasive materials to eliminate larger scratches or defects & replace them with smaller ones. Final finish of the composite surfaces is a result of the combination of filler particles size effects & finishing scratches. Polishing produces very little cutting but does tend to smear material from remaining high spots & create a smooth surface.

Polishing

The contoured restoration is done with very fine polishing discs, fine rubber points or cups &or composite polishing pastes.

Facial areas

Flame-shaped carbide finishing bur or polishing diamond is recommended for removing excess composite. Medium speed with light intermittent brush strokes & an air coolant is used for contouring. Final finishing & polishing are achieved with a rubber polishing point & sometimes, an aluminium oxide polishing paste.

For some areas: Commercially available abrasive discs mounted on a mandrel specific to disc type,in an angle handpiece at low speed,can be substituted for or used after the finishing bur or diamond.

Lingual areas

A round or oval 12-carbide finishing bur or diamond at medium speed with air coolant and light intermittent pressure. White stones in various shapes and sizes also may be used for final finishing of lingual surface,

Proximal and embrasure areas

Should be assessed visually and tactilely with an explorer and dental floss. A sharp gold finishing knife,amalgam knife or no.12 surgical blade mounted in a BP-handle well suited for removing excess material from the gingival proximal area. The instrument should be moved from the tooth to the restoration or along the margins, using light shaving strokes, keeping a portion of the cutting edge on the external enamel surface as a guide to prevent overreduction. The curved shape of the no.12 blade and the thin diameter makes it ideal for removing gingival overhangs.

Further contouring & finishing of proximal surfaces can be completed with abrasive finishing strips as well. Some strips have two different types of abrasives – medium and fine; on opposing ends of the strip, with a small area between where no abrasive is present to allow easy and safe insertion of the strip through the contact area. The medium grit is usually zirconium silicate & the fine grit is generally aluminium oxide. Diamond coated thin metal strips are also commercially available. The strip should be curved over the restoration & tooth surface

Occlusion

Rubber dam is removed if it was used. The patient is asked to close lightly on a piece of articulating paper & slide the mandibular teeth over the restored area. If excess present, small amounts at a time is removed and rechecked with articulating paper. Sometimes adjacent & / or opposing natural teeth need to be recontoured, care to be taken to avoid injudicious removal of too much tooth structure or restorative material.

L.Q.A.11 Porcelain bonded to metal ?

Ans. Metal ceramic restorations are the porcelain fused to metal (PFM) or the metal bonded restorations. This is advantageous as the restoration has a good fit of metal casting & esthetics of porcelain.

TYPES OF METAL CERAMIC SYSTEMS

Cast metal ceramic restoration

- Cast noble metal alloys (feldspathic porcelain)
- Cast base metal alloys (feldspathic porcelain)
- Cast tilanium (ultra low fusing porcelain)

Swaged metal ceramic restorations

- Gold alloy foil coping.
- Bonded platinum foil coping.

Ideal requirements

- CTE of alloy should be close or nearly the same as that of porcelain.
- The fusion temperature of the alloy should be higher than that of porcelain so that it does not melt or sag at the firing temperature.
- It should have a high modulus of elasticity to prevent flexing of metal framework & hence avoid fracture of porcelain.
- It should be capable of forming a bond with porcelain. The
- Composition should provide constituents for oxide formation which provide a chemical bond with porcelain. The alloy should be capable of wetting while porelain is applied to it & hence aid in mechanical bonding.
- It should not contain copper or silver as they stain in the interface & discolour porcelain.
- It should have a high proportional limit to avoid excess stress on the porcelain. Which is brittle.

Compositions

Of alloys:

- Should include platinum, palladium, which increases fusion temperature & reduce CTE.
- Should contain zinc, tin indium, chromium which form the surface oxide layer for chemical bonding of porcelain.

Of ceramics for PFM:

- The alkali content of porcelain is increased.
- Increases in the quatity of soda & potash increases the CTE to match that of the metal to which it is fused.
- But increased alkali content gives a tendency to devitrify porcelain & appear cloudy.
- For masking the colour of metal, opacifiers are added.

	Dentin porcelain	Enamel porcelain
Silica (siO2)	59.2	63.5
Alumina (Al2 O3)	18.5	18.9
Soda (Na2O)	4.8	5.0
Potash (K2O)	11.8	2.3
Boric oxide (B2O3)	4.6	0.12
Zinc oxide (ZNO)	0.58	0.11
Zirconium oxide (ZaO2)	0.39	0.13

Sample percentage composition of porcelain powder-

Comprises of one typical kit-

- Enamel porcelain powders in various shades (in bottles)
- Dentin porcelain powders in various shades (in bottles) Liquid foe mixing enamel dentin, gingival & transparent.
- Opaquer powders in various shades /together with a liquid for mixing.
- Gingival porcelain powder in various shades
- Transparent porcelain powder.
- A variety of stain (color) powders.

- Glaze powder
- Special liquid for mixing stains & glaze.

L.Q.A.12 Direct filling gold ?

Ans. It's a unique characteristic of gold to be welded at room temperature – (cold welded makes it possible for use of gold as a direct filling material into prepared cavities.

The types of direct filling gold are –

Foil

- Sheet.
  - Cohesive.
  - Non cohesive
- Ropes
- Cylinders
- Laminated
- Platinized.

Electrolytic precipitate (Mat gold)

- Mat
- Mat foil
- Alloyed

Gold foil

It is the oldest of all products manufactured – gold is malleable, so only one softening heat treatment (annealing) is required in beating a cast ingot of 15 mm thickness to a sub-microscopic thickness of 15-25 mm. The product is called *'Gold foil"*.

The crystals of the original cast metal are deformed & elongated so that they have a fibrous structure.

Supplied as

Flat square sheets of varying thickness.

- No. 4 wt. 4 grains (0.259 gm) 0.51 mm thick
- No. 3 wt 4 grains (0.194 gm) 0.38 mm thick

No. 3 gold foil is used in the manafacture of electrolytic & powder products.

- These sheets may be cut into 8th, 16th, 64th, etc. & then compressed into pellets or cylinders.
- A number of sheets of foil may be placed on top of each other. To form laminated gold foil a sheet of pure platinum foil is sandwiched between 2 sheets of pure gold foil.
- The foils can also be made into preformed cylinders & ropes.

Cohesive and noncohesive gold

All forms of direct filling gold could be supplied in cohesive & non cohesive conditions, they may be classified as being cohesive, semicohesive & non cohesive.

- The gold essentially free of surface contaminants are called cohesive gold foils.
- The ammonia treated foil is called non - cohesive foil.

Preformed foils

Ropes & cylinders are available.

Both are made form No.4 that has been "carbonized" or ";corrugated"

By placing the gold foil in between sheets of paper & igniting it in a closed container corrugated foil can be obtained. On igniting, the paper gets charred but the gold foil is left unharmed except that it becomes corrugated: this is because of the shriveling of the paper while oxidizing in air – tight safe.

Platinized Foil

- This might be considered a laminated foil in which pure platinum foil is sandwiched between two sheets of pure gold foil.
- The layers of platinum & gold are bonded together by a "cladding" process during the rolling operation.
- This increases the hardness of the restoration.
- Its available only in No 4 sheet form.

Electrolytic precipitate

It crystalline gold powder formed by electrolytic precipitation. the powder is formed into shapes or strips by sintering. It can be available as *MAT,*

Mat foil & alloyed

Mat gold

- These are formed into strips. These strips can be cut into the desired size by the operator.
- Its easy to build up the internal bulk of the restoration, as it can be more easily compacted & adopted to the cavity.
- Gold foil is recommended for the external surface of the restoration. Thus the mat gold is covered with a veneer of foil.
- If it is used directly on the surface there are chances of voids, because the crystalline form of mat powder doesn't permit easy welding into a solid homogenous mass.

Mat foil

Is a sandwich of electrolytic precipitated gold powder between sheets of No. 3 gold foil.

The sandwich is sintered & cut into strips of differing widths; which can be cut into desired lengths,

Alloyed electrolytic precipitate

The newest form of electrolytic gold is an alloy of gold & calcium called electroly RV. For greater ease of handling, the alloy is sandwiched between 2 layers of gold foil.

Calcium produces stronger restorations by dispersion strengthening, which locks in cold work strengthening. Alters the crystalline structure. So that the hardness & strength will be increased.

Powder gold

Chemically precipitated gold powders have been available in agglomerated form.

These agglomerates were usually a furnished with a liquid such as alcohol or dil, carbolic acid which held the agglomerate together, until its compacted. But the agglomerates usually disintegrated during compation., so the gold powder was enclosed in No. 3 gold foil.

A fine powder is formed by chemical precipitation or by atomizing the metal. the pellets (a blend of various particle sizes), is mixed with wax (which is later burnt of) and then wrapped with gold foil (No. 3)

The foil acts as an effective container for the powdered metal & acts as a matrix throughout the mass while its condensed.

The powdered gold pellets have a cylindrical or irregular shape & a diameter of 1-2 mm. The ratio ofgold foil to powder varies from 1 : 3 for the smallest pettets to approx 1 : 9 for the largest.

Degassing or desorbing

During storage & packaging, the direct filling golds are exposed to the atomsphere gas can adsorb on the surface of the gold. So its necessary to head the foil or pellet immediately before it's carried into the prepaced camity.

This heating process which removes surface gases & ensures a clean surface is called desorbing or degassing.

Desorbing is essential to remove the surface gases (oxygen nitrogen, ammonia, moisture or sulphur dioxide).

Direct filling golds may be heated by one of 2 methods.

- In bulk on a tray by gas – flame or electricity
- Piece by piece, in a well – adjusted alcohol flame.

In practice all but the powder gold may be desorbed on a tray heated electrically. Powder gold must be heated in a flame to ensure the complete burning away of wax ELECTRIC ANNEALING.

The electric "annealer" is maintained at a temperature between 340°C - 370°C the time required varies from 5-20 mins depending on the temperature & the quantily of gold on the tray.

Flame desorption

Each piece is picked indiuidually, heated directly in the open flame & placed in the prepared cavity. the fuel for the flame may be alcohol or gas-alcohol – pure methanol or ethanol without elorants or other additives.

Advantages

- Ability to select a piece of gold of the desered size
- Desorption of only those piece used.
- Less exposure to contaminations between time of degassing & use.
- Less danger of oversintering.

S.Q.A.1 Original gamma phase ?

Ans. The original gamma phase in amalgam alloys & set dental amalgams has a stoichiometry formula of Ag3Sn, the silver-tin system. In the range of composition around gamma phase, increases or decreases in silver influence the amounts of beta (low copper) & gamma phases & the properties.

If the tin concentration exceeds 26.8 wt%, a mixture of gamma phase & a tin-rich phase is formed. The presence of the tin phase increases the amount of tin-mercury phase is formed when the alloy is amalgamated. The tin-mercury phase lacks corrosion resistance & is the weakest component of the dental amalgam. Amalgams of tin-rich alloys display less expansion than do silver-rich alloys. Ag-Sn alloys are quite brittle & difficult to comminute uniformly unless a small amount of copper is substituted for silver.

The physical properties of the hardened amalgam depend on the relative percentages of each of the microstructural phases. The unconsumed Ag-Sn particles have a strong effect. The more this phase that is retained in the final structure, the more stronger is the amalgam. Generally, Ag3Sn phases are stable in an oral environment. The interface between the gamma phase & the matrix is important. The high proportion of the unconsumed gamma phase does not strengthen the amalgam unless the particles are bound to the matrix.

S.Q.A.2 Mercury toxicity

Ans. It is still sometimes conjectured that mercury toxicity from dental restorations is the cause for certain undiagnosed illnesses & that a real hazard may exist for the dentist or dental assistant when mercury vapor is inhaled during mixing, placement, & removal.

Undoubtedly, mercury penetrates from the restoration into tooth structure. An analysis of dentin underlying amalgam restorations reveals the presence of mercury, which in part may account for discoloration of the tooth. Use of radioactive mercury in silver amalgam has also revealed that some mercury might even reach the pulp. Small amounts of mercury are released during mastication. However, the possibility of toxic reactions occurring in patients from these traces of mercury penetrating the tooth or sensitization from mercury salts dissolving from the surface of the amalgam is rare.

The most significant contribution to mercury assimilation from dental amalgam is via vapor phase. The patient's encounter with mercury vapor during insertion is brief, & the total amount released during function is far below the 'no effect' level. Dentists and their auxillaries are exposed daily to the risk of mercury intoxication.although metallic mercury can be absorbed through the skin or by ingestion, the primary risk to dental personnel is from inhalation. The potential hazards of mercury can be greatly reduced by attention to a few precautionary measures. First, the operatory should be well-ventilated. All excess mercury, including waste, disposable capsules, & amalgam removed during condensation, should be collected & stored in well-sealed containers. Proper disposal through reputable dental vendors is mandatory to prevent environmental pollution. Amalgam scrap & materials contaminated with mercury or amalgam should not be incinerated or subjected to heat sterilization. If mercury is spilled, it must be cleaned immediately. If mercury comes in contact with the skin, it should be immediately washed with soap & water.

An important part for handling toxic materials is periodic monitoring of actual exposure levels & can be conducted annually. Film badges are also available that can be worn by office personnel in a manner similar to radiation exposure badges.

S.Q.A.3 Marginal leakage of restorations ?

Ans.

Microleakage

Dental amalgam has a good record of clinical performance, because of its tendency to minimize marginal leakage.

Self – sealing

The corrosion products of amalgam formed as it ages, sealed the interface (tooth – restoration & thereby prevent leakage - Hence a self - sealing restoration.

Because the brittle amalgam margins are unsupported in cases with delayed expansion or protruding restorations, they are susceptible to fracture & marginal defects resulting in leakage. Leakage can produce marginal discoloration with further corrosion & pitting caused by the concentration cells formed. This reduces the strength & may crumble under stress.

Cyclic ingress & egress of fluids at the restoration margin is called percolation. Percolation along the margins of an amalgam restoration is due to its difference in linear co-efficient of thermal expansion from tooth structure during intra – oral temperature changes.

Fluid influx occurs during cooling (contraction)

Fluid efflux occurs during heating (expansion) heat flow through a material is measured in terms of either the relative rate of heat conduction (thermal conductivity) be the amount of heat conduction per unit time (thermal diffusivity).

S.Q.A.4 Cavity varnish ?

Ans. Is a solution of one or more resins which when applied onto the cavity walls, evaporates leaving a thin resin film that serves a barriers between the restoration & the dentinal tubules.

Composition

Natural gum such as copal rosin or synthetic resin dissolved is an organic solvent such as alcohol acetone or ether.

- Medicinal agents such as chlorbutanol, thymol & eugenol may be added.
- Fluorides may also be added.

Manipulation

- A brush wire loop or a small pledget of cotton is used to apply.
- Several thin layers are applied each layer allowed to dry before the next.
- A uniform & continous coating in attained.

Uses

- It reduces microleakage around margins of newly placed amalgam, reduces postoperative sensitivity,
- It reduces passage of irritants into dentinal tubules from overlying restoration or base
- Prevent penetration of corrosion products into dentinal tubules in amalgam – prevents discoloration.
- May be used as surface coating over certain restoration to avoid dehydration or contact with oral fluids e.g. Silicate & GIC.
- May be applied on surface of metallic restoration as a temporary protection in galvanic shock.
- In cases where electrosurgery is to be done adjacent to a metallic restoration, varnish acts as a Temporary electrical insulator.

S.Q.A.5 Bonding agents

Ans. Bonding agents are described in two ways:

1. Enamel bond agents
2. Dentin bond agents

Enamel bond agents

Since the composite resins are more viscous, they don't flow easily into the micoporosities of etched enamel. Thus, enamel bond agents developed enhance the wettability of etched enamel.

Composition: They are unfilled resins similar to that of the resin matrix of composite resin, diluted by other monomers to lower the viscosity.

Dentin bond agents

There is difficulty for resin bonding with dentin or cementum & these can't be acid etched, as it can injure the pulp, hence the dentin bonding agents used. Supplied as a kit containing primers / conditioners & the bonding liquid.

Dentin bonding agents are classified as

- First generation
- Second generation.

- Third generation.
- Fourth generation.
- Fifth generation.

Advantages

- Single step application
- Less technique sensitive as it can bond to moist dentin
- Less volatile liquid
- Pleasant odor
- Higher bond strength

Mode of bonding

Probably micromechanincal, due to the penetration of the polymerizable monomer into the finely textured primed dentin.

Indications

- Bonding composites to teeth
- Bonding composites to porcelain & various metals like amalgam, base metal & noble metal alloys.
- Desensitization of exposed dentin or root surface.
- Bonding of porcelain veneers.

S.Q.A.6 Composite restorative m terials ?

Ans. The term composite material may be defined as a compound of two or more distinctly different materials with properties that are superior or intermediate to those of the individual constituents. Composite resin is basically a resin which has been strengthened by adding silica particles.

Classification–I

According to size of filler

Coventional	8 – 12 mm
Small particle	1 – 5 mm
Microfilled	0.04 – 04 mm
Hybrid	0.6 – 1 mm

According to curing

- Chemically activated.
- Light activated.

Composition

Essentials		
Resin matrix / binder	:	BISGMA or urethane dimethacrylate
Filler	:	Quartz, colloidal silica or heavy metal glasses
Coupling agent	:	Organo silanes.
Also contains		
Hydroquinone	:	Inhibitor to prevent premature polymerization
UV absorbers	:	To improve color stability aluminium oxide
Color pigments	:	To match tooth color

Uses

- Restoration of anterior & posterior teeth (directly or as inlays)
- To veneer metal crowns & bridges.
- To build up cores
- Cementation of orthodontic brackets, Maryland bridges & ceramic crowns, inlays, onlays & laminates.
- Pit & fissure sealants
- Esthetics laminates
- Repair of chipped porcelain restorations

S.Q.A.7 Composition and properties of type-III gold ?

Ans. Type-III alloys are for inlays & onlays.

Role of each constituent

Gold: Provides tarnish & corrosion resistance & has a desirable appearance, Also provides ductility & malleability.

Copper: It is the principal hardner. It reduces the melting point & density of gold.

In sufficient quantity gives a reddish color. Also helps to age harden gold alloys. In greater amounts reduces resistance to tarnish & corrosion of the alloy (hence shouldn't be >16 %)

Silver : Whitens the alloy (counteracts the reddish color of copper)

- It increases strength & hardens slightly.
- In large amounts – reduces tarnish resistance.

Platinum: Increases strength & corrosion resistance:

- Also increases melting point & has a whitening effect on the alloy.
- Helps to reduce the grain size.

Palladium: Similar to platinum

- Hardens & whitens the alloy
- Also raises fusion temperature & provides tarnish resistance.
- Is less expensive than platinum thus cost effective alloy.

Minor additions

Zinc: Acts as a scavenger for oxygen.

Without zinc, the silver in the alloy causes absorption of oxygen during melting later during solidification, the oxygen in rejected producing gas porosities in the casting.

Indium, tin, and iron: Help to harden the ceramic gold – palladium alloys (iron most effective).

Gallium: Added to compensate for the decreased CTE (in silver – free alloy – used to reduce the tendency for green staining at the metal porcelain margin)

Iridium, ruthenium, rhenium: Help to decrease the grain size. Added in small quantities (about 100 – 150 mm)

S.Q.A.8 Advantages of polycarboxylate cement

Ans. This was the first cement system developed with potential for adhesion to tooth structure.

Uses

- Primarily for luting permanent restorations.
- As bases & liners.
- Used in orthodontics for cementation of bonds.
- Also used as rool canal fillings in endodontics.

S.Q.A.9 IRM

Ans.

Glass ionomer- Resin combination materials-

Composition: Contain compoments of both resin & glass ionomer.

Powder

- Ion leachable glasses (silica alumina)
- Photoinitiators or chemical initiators or both
- Polymerizable resin

Liquid

- Polyacrylic acid
- Water
- Methacrylate monomer
- Hydroxyethyl methacrylate monomers.

Properties

Strength: Slightly lower (105 Mpa) – compressive greater (20 Mpa) – tensile Hardness – 40 KHN

Adhesion: Similar to GIC

Micromechanical retention helps.

These bond better to composites.

Microleakage: Greater compared to GIC.Partly due to polymerization shrinkage & partly, reduced wetting of the tooth by the cement.

Anticariogenitity: Significant due to fluoride release.

Pulpal response: Is mild

Esthetics: Less translucent due to difference in refractive index between resin matrix & powder particles.

Manipulation

RMGI Is mixed & applied after conditioning the tooth with polyacrylic acid (10 – 25 %).

PMC is placed after phosphoric acid etching, bond agent application & light cured.

S.Q.A.10 What are the advantages & disadvantages of porcelain?

Ans. **Advantages**

- Are most suitable tooth colored restorative materials.
- Used to make denture teeth, Single unit crowns, FPD'S & labial veneers.
- Most durable esthetic material
- Impervious to oral fluids
- Biologically compatible.
- Chemically indistructible in most environment.

Disadvantages

- Brittle material
- Have low tensile strength & fracture to stresses.
- Higher compressive strength.

S.Q.A.11 Aluminous porcelain

Ans. Its alumina-reinforced porcelain its composition is similar to that of conventional porcelain except for the increased alumina content (40 – 50 %)

The dispersed alumina crystals strengthen the porcelain by interruption of crack propagation.

The crack, can't penetrate the alumina crystals as easily as it can glass.

Aluiminous porcelain is used to construct the core layer of the porcelain jacket crown. Conventional body & enamel porcelain is then condensed over & fired in the usual manner.

Aluuminous porcelain crowns are more esthetic, their strength is almost twice that of conventional & is suffiuient for use on anterior teeth.However, is inadequate for posterior teeth.

Is less expensive & require less removal of tooth sructure during tooth preparation.

S.Q.A.12 Dentine adhesives

Ans. There is difficulty for resin bonding with dentin or cementum & these can't be acid etched, as it can injure the pulp, hence the dentin bonding agents used. Supplied as a kit containing primers / conditioners & the bonding liquid.

Classification - Dentin bonding agents are classified as:

- First generation.
- Second generation.
- Third generation.
- Forth generation.
- Fifth generation.

Advantages

- Single step application
- Less technique sensitive as it can bond to moist dentin
- Less volatile liquid
- Pleasant odor
- Higher bond strength

Mode of bonding

Probably micromechanincal, due to the penetration of the polymerizable monomer into the finely textured primed dentin.

Indications

- Bonding composites to teeth

- Bonding composites to porcelain & various metals like amalgam, base metal & noble metal alloys.
- Desensitization of exposed dentin or root surface
- Bonding of porcelain veneers.

S.Q.A.13 Acid etch technique / acid etching

Ans. The acid etch technique is one of the most effective ways of improving the bond & marginal seal between resin & enamel.

It forms the basis for many other dental procedures like resin-bonded metal retainers porcelain laminate veneers & orthodontic brackets

Mode of bonding

- It creates microporosities by discrete etching of the enamel i.e. by selective dissolution of enamel rod centers or peripheries or both.
- It increases the surface area.
- Etched enamel has a high surface energy allowing resin to wet the tooth surface better & penetrate into the microporosities. When polymerized it forms *"resin tags"* which form a mechanical bond to the enamel.

Acid used - 37 % Phosphoric acid.

- Supplied as a colored get
- Brushes are used to apply or the acid is supplied in a syringe and an be dispensed onto the enamel

Procedure

- Clean & polish tooth with pumice
- Acid is then applied onto the enamel
- Initially was 60 secs, but now recommended - 15 secs.
- Rinse thoroughly with a stream of water for 15 secs.
- Thoroughly dry enamel
- Enamel should have a white frosted appearance
- Keep surface clean & dry & place resin

- Contamination with saliva (or blood) can prevent effective tag formation & severely reduce the bond strength.

S.Q.A.14 Convenience form

Ans. Convenience form is that shape or form of the preparation that provides for adequate observation, accessibility, & ease of operation in preparing & restoring the tooth.

On occasion, obtaining this form may necessitate extension of distal, mesial, facial, or lingual walls to gain adequate access to deeper portion of the preparation.

In preparations for gold foil, convenience form also includes establishing convenience points for starting of foil condensation, prepared by deepening, or making more acute, one or more point angles of the preparation.

The occlusal divergence of vertical (longitudinal) walls of tooth preparations for class II cast restorations also may be considered as convenience form. Extended proximal preparations beyond proximal contacts in another convenience form procedure.

S.Q.A.15 Pulp responses to glass ionomer cements

Ans. Pulpal response: mild

Type II – Relatively biocompatible.
Water settable cements show higher acidity.

Type I – More acidic than Type II (because of slower set & lower powder / liquid ratio)

4 Instruments and Equipment for Tooth Preparation

L.Q.A.1 Sharpening of hand instruments

Ans. Instruments with dull edges cause more pain, prolong operating time, are less controllable, & reduce quality & precision in tooth preparation. Hence, its essential that all instruments be sharp. Resharpening requires little time & is very rewarding.

Many types of sharpening equipment exist, including stationary sharpening stones, mechanical sharpeners, & stones that are used in handpiece.

Stationary sharpening stones

The most frequently used sharpening equipment consists of a block or stick of abrasive material called a 'stone'. The stone is supported on a firm surface & the instrument is oriented & held by hand while being stroked against the stone surface.stationary stones are often called 'oil-stones' because of the common practice of applying a coating of oil to them as an aid in sharpening process.

Stationary oil stones

Are available in coarse, medium, or fine grit. Only a fine grit is suitable for the final sharpening of dental instruments. Coarse & medium grits may be used for initial reshaping of a badly damaged instrument or for sharpening other dental equipment such as bench knives.

Stationary stones can be obtained in various shapes including flat, grooved, cylindric, & tapered. Flat stones – preferred for sharpening all instruments with curved cutting edged. Cylindric – for instruments with concave edges, & tapered – permit using portion of the stone with a curvature matching that of the instrument.

Sharpening stones are made from any of several natural or synthetic materials. 4 types of materials are in common use for sharpening stones: Arkansas stone, silicon carbide, aluminum oxide & diamond.

Arkansas: Naturally occurring mineral containing microcrystalline quartz & traditionally has been preferred for fine sharpening stones.

Silicon carbide: Widely used industrial abrasive. It is the most commonly used material for grinding wheels & sandpapers as well as sharpening stones.

Aluminum oxide: Is increasingly used to manufacture sharpening stones & are commonly produced in various textures from different particle sizes of abrasive.

Diamond: Is the hardest available abrasive & is most effective for cutting & shaping hard materials.

Mechanical sharpeners

Some dental personnel do not do enough hand sharpening to remain confident of their proficiency. Under such circumstances the use of a powered mechanical sharpener is of benefit.

Basically a mechanical sharpener moves a hone in a reciprocating motion at a low speed, while the instrument is held at an appropriate angulation & supported by a rest. Its easier than having to hold the instrument at the proper angulation while moving it relative to the hone.

Handpiece sharpening stones

Mounted SiC & aluminum oxide stones for use with both straight and angle handpieces are available in various sizes and shapes.

Basic principles of sharpening

- Sharpen only after they have cleaned and sterilized.
- Establish the proper bevel angle & the desired angle of the cutting edge to the blade before placing the instrument against the stone, & maintain these angles while sharpening.
- Use a light stroke or pressure against the stone to minimize frictional heat.

- Use a rest or guide whenever possible.
- Remove as little as possible from the blade.
- Lightly hone the unbeveled side of the blade after sharpening to remove the fine bur that may be created.
- After sharpening, resterilize the instrument along with other items on the instrument tray setup.
- Keep the sharpening stones clean and free of metal cuttings.

L.Q.A.2 Bur design

Ans. The term bur is applied to all rotary cutting instruments that have bladed cutting heads.

Function

- Dental burs are minature milling cutters as used in industry.
- Are available in varions sizes & shapes depending on the purpose of preparing, finishing cavities & restorations.

Classification

Classified according to their compostition:

- Made from hypereutectoid steel with hardening agent added in minor amount – carbon steel or steel burs.
- Tungsten carbide burs or carbide burs.

Shapes

Refers to the contour or silhouette of the head. The basic head shapes are round, inverted cone, pear, straight fissure & tapered fissure.

Sizes

Has also traditionally served as a code for head design. The original numbering system grouped burs by 9 shapes & 11 sizes. The ½ & ¼ designations were added later when smaller instruments were included in the system. All original bur designs had continuous blade edges. Later, when crosscut burs were found to be more effective for cutting dentin at low speeds, crosscut versions of many bur sizes were introduced. This modification was indicated by adding 500 to the number equivalent non-crosscut size. Thus, a no.57 with crosscut was designated no. 557.

The system changed rapidly thereafter, but where the numbers are still used, the designs & dimensions remain the same.

As available handpiece speeds increased, a new cycle of modification of bur sizes & shapes occurred.

As the effectiveness of small burs has increased, larger burs have been replaced by them in many procedures.

Three other major trends in bur design are discernible: reduced use of crosscuts, extended heads on fissure burs & rounding of sharp tip angles.

Bur Blade Design

Each blade has 2 sides, the rake face (toward the direction of cutting) & clearance face, & three important angles, the rake angle, the edge angle and the clearance angle.

The rake angle is the most important design characteristic of a bur blade.

The face of the bur tooth is at an angle to the redial line from the center to the cutting edge. The angle is known as RAKE ANGLE.

If the face is beyond or leading the radial line in reference to the direction of rotation the angle formed between the face & the radial line is called Negative rake angle.

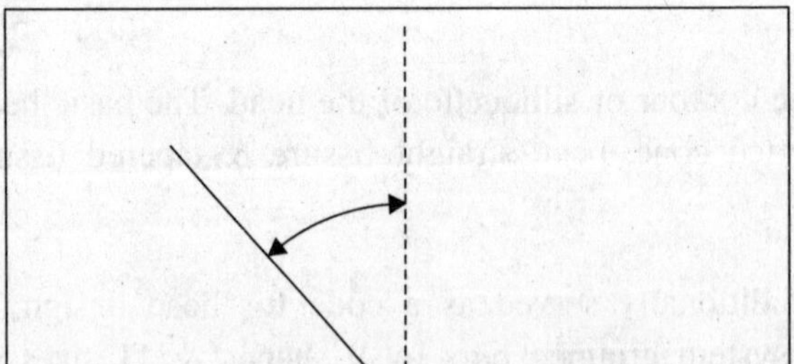

Negative rake angle

Where the radial line & the face contour correspond, the rake angle is zero. When the radial line leads the face so that the rake angle is on the inside of the radial line, is said to be positive rake angle.

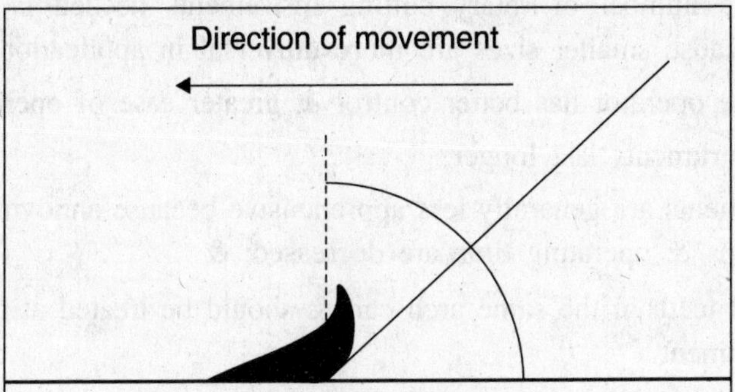

A rake angle is positive when the blade is behind the perpendicular

Clearance angle

Is the angle between the back of the tooth & the work is known as clearance angle. The plane surface immediately following the cutting edge is called the land. The angle it makes with the work is known as primary clearance. The angle between the back & the work is called secondary clearance.

S.Q.A.1 What is high speed ? Classify & describe its advantages and disadvantages ?

Ans. A high speed is a device for holding rotating instruments, transmitting power to them & for positioning them intra-orally. The rotational speed of an instrument is measured in revolutions per minute (rpm). Three speed ranges are generally recognized: low or slow speeds – below 12,000 rpm; medium or intermediate speeds - 12,000 to 200,000 rpm; & high or ultrahigh speeds – above 200,000 rpm. Most useful instruments are rotated at either low or high speed.

At high speed, the surface speed needed for efficient cutting can be attained with smaller & more versatile cutting instruments. This speed is used for tooth preparation & removing old restorations.

Advantages

- Diamond and carbide cutting instruments remove tooth structure faster with less pressure, vibration, & heat generation;
- The number of rotary cutting instruments needed is reduced because smaller sizes are more universal in application;
- The operator has better control & greater ease of operation;
- Instruments last longer;
- Patients are generally less apprehensive because annoying vibrations & operating time are decreased; &
- Several teeth in the same arch can & should be treated at the same appointment.

Variable control to regulate the speed makes the handpiece more versatile. This allows the operator to easily obtain the optimal speed for the size & type of rotating instruments at any stage of a specific operation.

Disadvantages

This type is usually avoided in procedures that require controlled application like caries removal & cavity preparation refinement. This is because, fine tactile discrimination is required in complete caries removal and hence high speed contraindicated. Though, a high speed handpiece using a round bur operated just above stall-out speed (low speed).

S.Q.A.2 Gingival marginal trimmer ?

Ans. A chisel-bladed instrument with the cutting edge in the plane of the instrument is termed a hatchet. The gingival marginal trimmer is a modified hatchet. Two distinct modifications of the basic hatchet design are observed. First, whereas the cutting edge of a hatchet is at a right angle to the axis of the blade, the cutting edge of a gingival marginal trimmer is at an angle other than a right angle to the axis of the blade.

Second, while the hatchet has a straight blade, the blade of the gingival trimmer is curved; hence termed is a double-plane instrument.

The curved blade accentuates the lateral scraping ability of the instruments. All double-plane instruments are lateral-cutting instruments.

These are paired instruments & are referred to as left & right. In addition, since this lateral-cutting instruments is used essentially for beveling gingival cavosurface margins, both distal & mesial trimmers are essential.

A typical distal GMT is designed to plane or bevel the cervical cavosurface margins of distal proximal amalgam & certain inlay preparations.

A typical mesial GMT is used to plane mesial cervical margins.

S.Q.A.3 Angle former

Ans. A chisel is an excavator primarily used for planing or cleaning enamel & dentin. An angle former is a modified chisel. The cutting edge of an angle former is sharpened at an angle to the axis of the blade. The blade of the cutting edge to the blade axis of the angle former is usually 80-85 centigrades.

Since the cutting edge of the angle former is not at right angle to the blade axis, a forth unit is incorporated into black's instrument formula. The number, which again takes the second position in the formula, indicates in centigrades the angle of cutting edge with the axis of the shaft.

The acute cutting angle being directed to the right or to the left makes the angle former always a paired instrument. An indented ring on the shaft or shank identifies the right of the pair.

Angle formers are used to accentuate line & point angles in the internal outline form in cavities for cohesive gold to establish retention form. The action of the instrument is essentially one of lateral scraping.

The blade of the angle former is beveled on the sides as well as the end to form 3 cutting edges. Beveling of the blade laterally, together with the end bevel, forms 3 distinct cutting edges. This triple cutting edge is frequently applied to chisel & hoes, particularly those of small dimension. The instrument loses none of its end-cutting quality that is very useful in shaping and refining.

S.Q.A.4 Coolants in dentistry

Ans. Most common instrument coolants are air or air-water spray. Air alone as a coolant is not effective in preventing pulpal damage because it needlessly desiccates the dentin & damages the odontoblasts. Air has a much lower heat capacity than water and is much less efficient in absorbing unwanted heat. An air coolant alone should be used only when visibility is a problem, such as during finishing procedures of tooth preparations. Air is applied only to the extent of removing excess moisture, leaving a glistening surface. At such times, air coolant combined with both lower speed & light intermittent application, should be used to enhance vision & minimize trauma. Air-water spray is universally used to cool, moisten & clear the operating site during normal cutting procedures. In addition, the spray lubricates, cleans, & cools the cutting instrument, thereby increasing its efficiency & service life. A well-designed & properly directed air-water spray also helps keep the gingival crevice open for better vision when gingival extension is necessary. The use of a water spray & its removal by an effective high-volume evacuator are especially important when old amalgam restorations are removed because they decrease mercury vapor release & increase visibility.

NOTES

5

Isolation of The Operating Field

L.Q.A.1 What is the importance of 'moisture control' in operative dentistry? Give different methods of controlling moisture during operative procedures?

Ans. The goals of operating field isolation are moisture control, retraction & harm prevention. Operative dentistry cannot be executed properly unless the moisture is controlled. For best results, operative procedures require adequate isolation of the operating field. Moisture control refers to excluding sulcular fluid, saliva, & gingival bleeding from the operating field. It also refers to preventing the hand piece spray & restorative debris from being swallowed or aspirated by the patient. The operator can best perform dental procedures like caries removal, proper tooth preparation & insertion of restorative materials in a dry field. Such preparations are less prone to post-operative problems related to contamination from oral fluids. Also, time is saved by operating in a clean field with good visibility. Thus, moisture control, contributes immensely to patient comfort & operator efficiency.

Methods

The rubber dam, suction devices, & absorbents are varyingly effective in moisture control. Generally, the rubber dam is the recommended technique for moisture control. Local anesthesia is also important in moisture control.

Rubber dam

Use of this ensures proper dryness of teeth & improves the quality of clinical restorative dentistry. It is used to define the operating field by isolating one or more teeth from the oral environment. The dam eliminates saliva from the operating site & retracts soft tissues. Plus there are fewer interruptions of replacing cotton rolls to maintain isolation.

Advantages

- A dry, clean operating field,
- Improved access and visibility
- Potentially improved properties of dental materials
- Protection of the patient & the operator
- Operating efficiency.

Cotton roll isolation & cellulose wafers: absorbents such as cotton rolls & cellulose wafers are alternatives when rubber dam application is impractical or impossible. They provide acceptable moisture control for most of the procedures. Using a saliva ejector in conjunction further abates salivary flow. Cotton rolls are placed in the vestibule of the operating site. Cellulose wafers may be used to retract the cheek & provide additional absorbency.

Saliva ejectors & high-volume evacuator

It removes saliva that collects on the floor of the mouth. It may be used in conjunction with sponges, cotton rolls, & rubber dam. Disposable, inexpensive plastic ejectors that may be shaped by bending with fingers are preferable because of improved infection control.

L.Q.A.2 Describe components of rubber dam kit

Ans.

Components of rubber dam kit

The materials & instruments necessary for the use of the rubber dam are available easily.

Material

Rubber dam material is available in 5 × 5 inch (12.5 × 12.5 cm) or 6 × 6 inch (15 × 15 cm) sheets. Sterile dam material is also available packaged as individual sheets. The thicknesses or weights available are thin (0.006 inch [0.15 mm]), medium (0.008 inch [0.2 mm]), heavy (0.010 inch [0.25 mm]), extra heavy (0.012 inch [0.30 mm]), & special heavy (0.014 inch [0.35 mm]).

Both light & dark dam materials are available, but the dark color is preferred for contrast. Green & blue color is also marketed. Rubber dam material has a shiny & a dull side. Because the dull side is less light reflective, it is generally placed facing the occlusal of the isolated teeth. Generally, dark, heavy, 6x6 inch sheets are recommended.

Holder

The rubber dam holder (frame) maintains the borders of the rubber dam in position. The Young holder is a U-shaped metal frame with small metal projections for securing the borders of the rubber dam. It is easily applied & comfortable for the patient. An optional adjustable neck strap may be placed behind the parient's neck & is attached to 2 hooks, 1 in the middle of each side of the frame. The neck strap is lightly tightened to snug the dam & frame to the face & maximize retraction & provide access to the operating site.

Retainer

The rubber dam retainer (clamp) consists of 4 prongs & 2 jaws connected by a bow. The retainer is used to anchor the dam to the most posterior tooth to be isolated. Retainers are also used to retract gingival tissue. Many different shapes and sizes are available, with specific retainers designed for certain teeth.

When positioned on a tooth, a properly selected retainer should contact the tooth in 4 areas – 2 on the facial surface & 2 on the lingual surface. This 4 point contact prevents rocking or tilting of the retainer.

Wingless & winged retainers are available. The wings are designed to provide extra retraction of the rubber dam from the operating field & to allow attachment of the dam to the retainer before conveying the retainer to the anchor tooth. The bow of the retainer should be tied with a dental floss approximately 12 inches in length before the retainer is placed in the mouth.

Punch

The rubber dam punch is a precision instrument having a rotating metal table (disk) with six holes of varying sizes & a tapered, sharp pointed plunger. The plunger should be centered in the cutting hole so the edges of the holes are not at a risk of being chipped by the plunger tip when the plunger is closed.

Retainer forceps

The rubber dam retainer forceps is used both for placement & removal of the retainer from the tooth.

Napkin

The rubber dam napkins are soft, absorbent, & disposable. Has following advantages:

- It prevents skin contact with rubber to reduce possibility of allergic reactions in sensitive patients
- It absorbs saliva seeping at the corners of the mouth.
- It acts as a cushion
- Provides a convenient method of wiping the patient's lips on removal of the dam.

Lubricants

A water soluble lubricant applied in the area of the punched holes facilitates the passing of the dam septa through the proximal contacts. A rubber dam lubricant is commercially available, but others like shaving cream or soap slurry, are also satisfactory. Cocoa butter or petroleum jelly may be applied to patient's mouth to prevent irritation (but are not satisfactory rubber dam lubricants as are oil based).

Modelling compound

Low-fusing compound is sometimes used to secure the retainer to the tooth to prevent retainer movement during the procedure.

Anchors (other than retainers)

May be used. Waxed dental tape, or a small piece of rubber dam material may be passed through the proximal contact, looped & passed through a second time.

S.Q.A.1 Gingival retraction ?

Ans. Retraction cord is often used for isolation & retraction in the direct procedures of treatment of accessible subgingival areas & in indirect procedures involving gingival margins.

When the rubber dam is not used, is impractical or is inappropriate, retraction cord, usually moistened with a noncaustic styptic may be placed in the gingival sulcus to control sulcular seepage &/or hemorrhage. Most brands are available with & without the vasoconstrictor epinephrine, which also acts to control sulcular fluids.

To achieve adequate moisture control, it should be used in conjunction with salivation control by virtue of profound anesthesia of all tissues of the operating site. A properly applied retraction cord improves access & visibility & helps prevent abrasion of gingival tissue during tooth preparation. It helps restrict excess restorative material from entering the gingival sulcus & provide better access for contouring & finishing the restorative material.

NOTES

NOTES

6 Amalgam Restoration for Class–II Cavity Preparation

L.Q.A.1 Discuss procedures for formulations of proper contacts and contours ?

Ans. For the proper reproduction, with a restorative material of the physio-anatomical features of teeth, two operative acts must preecede or acompany the restorative procedure and they are:

- Tooth (Teeth) movement and
- Matricing.

Tooth movement

It is the act of either separating the involved teeth from each other, bringing them closer to each other and / or changing their spatial position in one or more dimensions. This is done in order to facilitate the creation of a physiologically functional contact, contour and occluding anatomy in the restored tooth.

Objectives

- To bring drifted, titled or restored teeth to their indicated physiologic positions as a pre-requisite for proper reproduction of the proximal surfaces in restorative materials.
- To close space between teeth not amenable to closure by the contemplated restoration.
- To move teeth to another location, so that when restored, they will be in a position most physiologically acceptable by the periodontium.

- To move teeth occlusally or apically in order to make them restorable.
- To move teeth from a non-functional traumatically functional location.
- To move teeth to a position, so that when restored, they will be in the most esthetically pleasing situation.
- To move teeth in a direction and to a location to increase the diensions of available tooth structure for the resistance and retention forms of the contemplated restoration.
- To create a space sufficient for the thickness of the matrix bond interproximally. The space should be in addition to the mesio-distal dimension of the restoration, not at its expense. This is necessary to create a positive, tight contact.

It can also be used as convenience means for facilitating access to proximal cavity preparations, especially class III preparations. In addition, it can be used to detech proximal decay, to facilitate adequate polishing of the restoration's proximal surfaces and to remove foreign bodies impacted proximally that are not dislodgeable by floss or brushes.

Two principal methods of tooth movements are:

- Rapid or immediate tooth movement and
- Slow or delayed tooth movement.

Rapid or immediate tooth movement

Mechanical type of seperations, creates either proximal separation at the point of the seperator's introduction and / or improved closeness of the proximal surface opposite the point of the seperator's introduction.

Indications

Can be used preparatory to slow tooth movement or to maintain a space gained by slow tooth movement.

Rapid tooth movement can be done by

1. Wedge method

Separation is accomplished by the insertion of a pointed wedge-shaped device between the teeth in order to create tseparation at the point or closure on the opposite proximal side of the involved teeth. The more the wedge moves facially or lingually, the greater will be the separation.

Ellist seperator

Indicated for short duration seperation that does not necessitate stabilization. Its useful in examining proximal surfaces or in final polishing of restored contacts.

Wood or plastic wedges

These are irregularly shaped wedges, usually made of medicated wood or synthetic resin. In cross-section the base of the triangle will be in contact with the interdental papillae, gingival to the gingival margin of the proximal cavity. The two sides of the triangle should coincide with the corresponding two sides (mesial & distal) of the gingival embrasure. The apex of the triangle should coincide with the gingival start of the contact area.

The wedge is used in conjuction with matrices for inserting plastic restorative materials.

Functions of wedges are

- They assure the close adaptability of the matrix band to the tooth, gingival to the gingival margin of the preparation.
- They occupy the space designated to be the gingival embrasure, preventing the restorative material from impinging on it, thus assuring proper helath for the gingival interdental col (papillae).
- They define the gingival extent of the contact area as well as the facial and lingual embrasures, thereby assuring the health of the proximal periodontal tissues.
- They create some separation to compensate for the thickness of the matrix band and minor drifting of the teeth.
- They establish atraumatic retraction of the rubber dam and the gingiva from the gingival margin of the cavity preparation.
- They assure the immobilization of the matrix band against movement both facial-lingually and cervico-occlusally during insertion of the restorative material.
- They protect the interproximal gingival from unexpected trauma.

Although wedges are supplied in different sizes to suit different locations; the wedges should be trimmed to exactly fit each gingival embrasure.

Advantages

- Are easily cut and trimmed and they absorb water intraorally.
- Resin wedges is that they can be physically molded and bent to correspond with the configuration of the interdental col.

  For instantaneous separation of teeth during operative procedures in anterior teeth.

2. Traction method

Done with mechanical devices which engage the proximal surfaces of the teeth to be seperated by means of holding arms. E.g. are:

- Non-interfering true.
- Ferrier double-bow seperator.

Slow and delayed tooth movement

When teeth gave drifted and / or tilted considerably rapid movement of teeth to the proper position will in danger the PDL. Therefore, slow tooth movement, over a period of weeks, will allow proper repositioning of teeth in a physiologic manner.

Methods

- ***Separating wires:*** Thin piece of wire are introduced gingival to the contact then wrapped around the contact area. The 2 ends are twisted together to create seperation not to exceed 0.5 mm. The twisted ends are then bent into the buccal or lingual embrasure to prevent impingement upon soft tissue or interference with food flow. The wires are then tightened periodically to increase the separation.
- ***Oversized tempories:*** Resin temporaries that are oversized mesio-distally may achieve slow seperation. Resin is added to the on tact areas periodically to increase the amount of separation, which will not exceed 0.5 mm per visit.

Matricing

Is the procedure whereby a temporary wall is created opposite to axial walls, surrounding areas of tooth structure that were lost during preparation. It is used with restorative materials that are introduced in a plastic state.

The matrix wall should possess the exact 3-dimensional contours of the future restoration and should be capable of imparting this configuration to the inserted restorative material during its plastically deformable state. Should be immobile during setting of the material and should not reach with or adhere to the material.

It should be easily removed after the material hardens without compromising the created contact and contour.

The matrix is formed of 2 parts:

- Band piece of metal or polymeric material to support and give form to the material during its introduction and hardening.
- The retainer band can be retained in its designated position and shape.

The matrix is essential for the proper reproduction of the proximal, facial and lingual anatomy in any restoration of plastic nature.

Types of matrices

Matrices for class I cavity preparatin to revieve a restorative material inserted in a plastic state.

Matrices for class II to revieve material in a plastic state:

- Single-banded tofflemire for class II designs 1, 2, 3, 6, 7, 8 preparations.
- Ivory matrix no. 1.
- Ivory matrix no. 8.
- Black's matrix i.e.-
  - For simple cases,
  - With a gingival extension.
- Soldered band or seamless copper band matrix.
- The anatomical matrix.
- Roll in band matrix (auto-matrix)

Matrices for a cavity preparation for amalgam restorations on the distal of te cuspid:

- S-shaped matrix.
- For a cavity preparation with incisal access on the distal of the cuspid the regular tofflemire could be used efficiently.

Matrices for class-III direct tooth colored restorations:

- For class-III in normal alignment of teeth.
- In irregular alignment.
- For two small proximal preparations in contact with each other.

Matrice for class-IV for direct tooth colored materials:

- Plastic strip for inciso-proximal.
- Aluminum foil incisal corner matrix.
- Transparent crown form matrices.
- Anatomic matrix.
- Modified S-shaped.

Matrices for class V amalgam:

- Window matrix.
- S-shaped.

Matrices for class-V preparations for direct tooth colored restorations:

- Anatomic matrix for non-light cured, direct tooth colored.
- Aluminium or copper collars for non-light cured, direct tooth colored.
- Anatomic matrix for light and non-light curved, direct tooth colored restorations.

Extra-oral formulations

The procedure is facilitated and made convenient through wax pattern and cast adjustments.

Wax pattern

Usually buit in a slightly overcontoured condition, especially at the contact area to allow for the finishing and polishing surface losses.

Removable dies make the procedure very feasible as they will allow addittions or removal of small increments of waxes at or from indirected areas.

Cast adjustments

Usually done with rubbery stones incrementally removing cast material surface to obtain the exact dimensions, configurations and interrelationship of the contact and contours.

L.Q.A.2 Discuss the retention and resistence form in Black's class-II restoration ?

Ans. Retention form

Retention form preparation features lock or retain the restorative material in the tooth. For nonbonded and bonded amalgam restorations, the amalgam must be mechanically locked inside the tooth.

Amalgam retention form is provided by:

- Mechanical locking of the inserted amalgam into surface irregularities of the preparation to allow good adaptation of the amalgam.
- Preparation of vertical walls that converge occlusally.
- Special retention features such as locks, grooves, cones, slots, pins, steps or amalgan pins that are plated during final stage of tooth preparation.
- Bonding of the amalgam to the tooth: The 1st and 2nd are considered primary retention form features and are provided by the orientation and type of the preparation instrument.
- The remaining two are secondary retention form features.

Primary retention form for class II cavity preparations is provided by the occlusal connergence of facial and lingual walls and by the dovetail design of the occlusal step.

Ideally secondary retention form for the occlusal and proximal portions of the preparation should be independent of each other.

To enhance retention form of the proximal portion, proximal locks may be indicated to counter proximal displacement.

There are four characteristics or determinants of proximal locks:

- Position.
- Translation.
- Depth.
- Occlusogingival orientation.

Position: The axicofacial and axiolingual line angles of initial tooth preparation.

Translation: The direction of movement of the axis of the bur.

Depth: The intent of translation.

Occlucogingival: The tilt of the bur, whuch dustate the occlusal height if the lock, given a constant depth.

Resistance form

Features help the restoration and tooth resist fracturing as a result of occlusal forces. Resistance features that assist in preventing the tooth from fracturing includes:

- Maintaining as much unprepared tooth structure as possible.
- Having pulpal and gingival walls prepared prependicular to occlusal forces.
- Having rounded internal preparatin angles.
- Removing unsupported or weakened tooth structure.
- Placing pins into the tooth as part of the final stage of tooth preparation.
- Bonding the amalgam in the tooth.

The last 2 of these are considered and secondary resistance form.

Resistance form features that preventing the amalgam from fracturing includes:

- Adequate thickness of amalgam.
- Marginal amalgam of 90° or greater.
- Box like preparation form, which provides uniform amalgam thickness.
- Rounded axiopulpal line angles in class II preparation.

Primary resistance for class II form is provided by:

- Pulpal and gingival walls being flat and perpendicular to forces directed with long axis of the tooth.
- Restricting extensions of the walls to allow strong cusps and ridge areas to remain with sufficient dentin support.
- Restricting the occlusal outline form to areas receiving minimal occlusal contact.

- The reserve curve optimizing the strength of both amalgam and tooth structure.
- Slightly rounding the intermal line angles to reduce stress concent ratio in tooth structure.
- Providing enough thickness of restorative material to prevent its fracture under mastication.

Secondary resistance form in final tooth preparation involves both resistance of the remaining tooth structure against fracture from oblique forces and resistance of restorative material against fracture.

L.Q.A.3 Define cavity, cavity preparation and prepared cavity ? Discuss preparation of a class II mesio-occlusally on a permanent mandibular first molar for amalgam ?

Ans. Cavity

The term cavity is used only as a historical reference. In the past, the term cavity was used to describe a carious lesion in a tooth that had progressed to the point that part of the tooth structure had been destroyed. Thus, the tooth was cavitated - a breach in the surface integrity of the tooth and hence referred to as a cavity.

Cavity preparation

When the affected tooth was repaired, the cutting or preparation of the remaining tooth structure to best revieve a restorative material was referred to as a cavity preparation.

The preparation of the tooth is no longer referred to as a "cavity preparation" but as "tooth preparation". Tooth preparation is defined as the mechanical alteration of a defective, injured, or diseased tooth to best revieve a restorative state of the tooth, including esthetic corrections where indicated, along with normal form and function.

Class-II amalgam restorations for mesio-occlusal tooth preparation on a mandibular 1st molar

1. Initial Tooth Preparation

Occlusal outline form (Occlusal step): The occlusal outline for, of a class-II tooth preparation for amalgam is similar to that for the class I tooth preparation.

Using high speed with air water spray, the mesial pit with a punch cut. The but should be rotating when applied to the tooth and should be rotating when applied to the tooth and should not step rotating until removed from the proximal and lingual (Facial) aspects, the long axis of the bur and the long axis of the tooth crown should remain parallel during cutting procedures. Maintaining it in this position, facial, lingual and distal walls with a slight occlusal convengence, which provides favourable amalgam angles at the margins.

Before rxtending into the involved mesial marginal ridge, the final location of the facial and lingual walls of the proximal box relative to the contact area, needs to be visualized.

A reverse curve in occlusal outline is usually created when mesio-facial enamel wall is parallel to enamel rod direction. Lingually, reverse curve is very slight, often unnecessary, because the imbrassure form is larger.

While maintaining the established pulpal depth and with the but parallel to the long axis if the tooth crown, extend the preparation mesially, stopping approx. 0.8 mm short of cutting through the marginal ridge into the contact area. The occlusal step in this region is made slightly wider faciolingually than in class I because additional width is necessary for the proximal box. This extension includes part of the mesial marginal ridge and exposes the marginal-ridge DEJ. The location of the DEJ is an important guide in the development of the proximal preparation.

- **Proximal outline form (proximal box)**

The objectives for extension of proximal margin are to:

- Includes all caries, faults or existing restorative material.
- Create 90°, cavo surface margins i.e. butt joint margins.
- Establish not more than 0.5 mm clearance with the adjacent proximal surface facially, lingually and gingivally.

The initial procedure in preparing the outline form of the proximal box is the isolation of the mesial enamel by the proximal ditch cut.

With the same orientation of the bur, positioned over DEJ in the pulpal floor next ot the remaining mesial marginal ridge, the end of the but cuts a ditch gingivally along the exposed DEJ, 2nd and 3rd at the expenses of dentin and one third at the expense of enamel. Approximately, 0.5-0.6 mm is cut into the dentin and 0.2-0.3 mm into enamel. Pressure is directed gingivally and lightly toward the mesial surface, while the bur is moved facially and lingually along the DEJ.

Clearance of proximal margins greater than 0.5 mm is excessive unless indicated to include caries, undermined enamel or existing restorative material.

The facial and lingual limits of the ditch should have a clearance of only 0.2-0.3 mm with the adjacent tooth.

The finished gingival margin should clear the adjacent tooth by only 0.5 mm (in a small preparation).

The proximal ditch cut should be sufficiently deep into dentin that retention locks, can be prepared into the axiolingual and axiofacial line angles without undermining the proximal enamel.

The proximal ditch cut mat be diverted gingivally to ensure that the faciolingual dimension at the gingival is greater than at the occlusal. It contributes to the retention form.

Final tooth preparation

Includes removal of any remaining defective enamel and infected carious dentin.

Any old restorative material remaining should not be removed if no evidence of recurrent caries.

Pulp protection is provided if the need arises.

Finishing external walls

The preparation walss and margins should not have unsupported enamel and marginal irregularities. Less marginal leakage occurs of the margins are straight and smooth.

Ideally, a 90° cavo surface bevel is indicated in the preparation.

The occlusal line angle may be 90 to 100° or greater.

Amalgam is a brittle material and may feature under occlusal stress ir its angle at the margin is less than 80°.

Finally, the preparation is cleaned and inspected.

The preparation may need desensitizing and bonding; just as in a class I preparation.

S.Q.A.1 Describe in detail conservative class-II preparation for amalgam in maxillary mesio-occlusal tooth

Ans. The MO tooth preparation is generally uncomplicated. Extension into the enamel oblique ridge is avoided whenever possible to maintain the cross-splinting strength it provides to the tooth. Occasionaly extension through the ridge and into the distal pit is necessary because of the extent of caries. The outline of this OL pit-and-fissure portion is similar to that of the class I, OL preparation.

When the occlusal fissure extends into the facial cusp ridge and it cannot be removed by enameloplasty, the defect should be eliminated by extension.

Occasionally, this can be done by tilting the bur to create an occlusal divergence of the facial wall. If this fault cannot be eliminated without extending the margin to the height of the cusp ridge or undermining enamel margin, extend the preparation facially through the ridge. The pulpal wall of this facial extension may have remaining enamel margin but a depth of 1.5 - 2 mm is necessary to provide sufficient bulk of material for adequate strength.

For best esthetic results, minimal extension of the proximal mesiofacial margin is indicated.

S.Q.A.2 Universal matrix retainer

Ans. The universal matrix system is ideally indicated when 3 surfaces i.e. mesial, occlusal, distal) of a posterior tooth have been prepared. Also called Tofflemire matrix retainer. It is commonly used also for the two surface class-II restoration. A definite advantage is that it may be positioned on the facial, or lingual aspect of the tooth.

The retainer and the band are generally stable when in place. The retainer is easily separated from the band to expedite removal of the band.

Bands of various occlusogingival widths are available. A small Tofflemire retainer is available for use with the primary dentition.

The conventional, flat band must be shaped (i.e. burnished) to achieve proper contour and contact.

The uncontoured bands are available in 2 thickness - 0.002 & 0.0015 inch. Much less time is required for placement of the Tofflemire matrix.

Preventoured bands are commercially available and need little or no adjustment before placing the retainer. These are simpler to use as they usually require little or no adjustment or modification after positioning around the tooth.

To prepare the retainer to receive the band, the larger of the knurled nuts is turned counterclockwise until the locking vise is a short distance (6 mm) from the retainer. Next, while holding the large nut, the smaller nut is turned counter clockwise until the pointed spindle is free of the slot in the locking vise. The matrix band is then folded end to end, forming a loop. Position the band in the retainer so that the slotted size of the retainer is directed gingivally to permit easy separation of the retainer. The 2nd ends of the band are placed in the slot of the locking vise, andthe smaller of the knurled nuts is turned clockwise to tighten the pointed spindle against the band. Next, turn the larger knurled nut clockwise to tighten the band slightly. Once the band is correctly positioned, tighten the band securely around the tooth.

S.Q.A.3 Automatrix ?

Ans. It is a retainerless matrix system with 4 types of bands that are designed to fit all teeth, regardless of circumference and height. The bands vary in height from 3/16 to 5/16 inch and are supplied in 2 thicknesses 0.0015 and 0.002 inch.

The indicated use of this matrix is for extensive class II preparations, especially those replacing two or more cusps.

One major advantage is that auto-lock lopp can be positioned either on the facial or lingual surface with equal case.

A major disadvantage is that the bands are not precontoured and development of physiologic proximal contours is difficult.

Advantages

- Convenience.
- Improved visibility as retainer absent.
- Ability to place the outlock loop on the facial or lingual tooth surface.
- Decreased time for application as compared to copper band matrix.

Disadvantages

- Band is flat and difficuly to burnish and is sometimes unstable even when wedges are in place.
- Development of proper proximal contours and contacts can be difficult.

S.Q.A.4 Smear layer

Ans. Whenever dentin has been cut or abraded, with rotary instruments,a thin altered layer is created on the surface & compacted unavoidably into a layer. This smear layer is only a few micrometers thick & is composed of denatured collagen, hydroxyapatite, & other cutting debris. The smear layer serves as a natural bandage over the cut dentinal surface because it occludes many of the dentinal tubules with debris called smear plugs. This creates a sealing, although it is 25-30 % porous. While the smear layer is a good protective barrier, it has relatively weak attachment to the dentin and is subject to dissolution by acids. Because it is partially porous, it cannot prevent slow long-term diffusion.

For unbonded amalgam restorations, enamel & dentin smear layers are left in place.

7

Pins in Restoration

L.Q.A.1 Give indications for pins in restoration ? Briefly describe the technique ?

Ans.

Indications

Use of pins (Complex posterior amalgam restorations) may be considered when large amounts of tooth structure are missing, when one or more cusps need copping and when increased resistance and retention forms are needed. They may be used as:

- Control restorations in teeth with questionable pulpal and / or periodontal prognosis;
- Control restorations in teeth with quite and severe caries.
- Definitive final restorations; or
- Foundations.

When determining the appropriateness of such restorations (pin-retained etc), following factors must be considered:

Resistance and retention forms

In a tooth severely involved with caries or existing restorative material, any undermined enamel or weak tooth structure subject to failure must be removed and restored.

In such selected cases, preparations may be designed for amalgam that improve the resistance form of a tooth.

When conventional retention fratures are nor adequate because of insufficient remaining tooth structure, pins, slots and amalgam bonding techniques may be used to enhance retention form; (depending on the amount of tooth structure remaining and the tooth being restored)

Pins, slots and bonding also provide additional resistance form to the restoration.

Status and Prognosis of the tooth

A tooth with severe caries that may require endodontic therapy or crown lengthening or that has an uncertain periodontal prognosis is often treated initially with a control restoration.

The status and prognosis of the tooth will determine the size, number and placement of retention features. Larger restorations generally requires more retention. Greater care needs to be taken in smaller teeth, in teeth that have been significantly excavated and in symptomatic teeth. Carelessness can risk pulpal irritation or exposure.

Role of tooth in the overall treatment plan

The restorative treatment choice for a tooth is influenced by its role in the overall treatment plan.

Use of complex restoration (pin, slots etc) is occasionally used as an alternative for indirect restorations. Other purposes are:

- Abutment teeth for fixed prosthesis need it as foundation.
- A tooth may be treated with complex restoration if adequate resistance and retention forms can be provided.
- For periodontal and orthodontic patients, its the restoration of choice until the final phase of treatment (when cast restorations may be preferred).

Occlusion, esthetics and economics

Complex restorations are indicated as interim restorations for teeth that require elaborate occlusal alterations ranging from vertical dimension changes to correcting occlusal plane discrepancies.

When cost of the restorations is a major factor for the patient, complex restorations is an appropriate treatment option.

Age and health of the patient

For some geriatric and debilitated patients, the complex restoration may be treatment of choice over more expensive and time-consuming cast restoration.

Clinical technique

Treatment options should be discussed with the patient.

Before the preparation for a complex amalgam restoration begins, an explanation of the procedure should be given to patient. The limitations of the restoration and the possible complications that might occur during the procedure also to be presented.

A pin hole retained restoration may be defined as any restoration requiring the placement of one or more pins in the dentin to provide adequate resistance and retention forms.

Pins are *used* whenever adequate resistance and retention forms cannot be established with slots, locks or undercuts only.

Pin-retained amalgam is an important adjunct in the restoration of teeth with extensive caries or fractures.

Is indicated in large class II restorations andalso in other types of large restorations. In class IV, rarely used. Because of the relatively small size of anterior teeth and the potential for enamel and dentin bonding, pins are rarely usedin anterior teeth or with composite restorative materials.

Occassionally, pins may be used for large class IV on the distal surface of a canine that involves a significant amount of the distoincisal corner.

Pins placed in the gingival portion may provide the needed retention for restoration. The use of pins may be considered for a tooth that has insufficient enamel present for acid-etching and / or insufficient remaining tooth structure for adequate retention features.Indications of pins in a class V is rare.

TOOTH PREPARATION

Initial

The initial preparation for the pin-retained complex amalgam restorations is similar to the conventional preparations of class-I or II cavity.

When caries is extensive, reduction of one or more of the cusps for capping may be indicated. When the facial or lingual extension exceeds 2/3rd the distance from a primary groove toward the cusp tip; reduction of the cusp(s) for amalgam is required for the development of adequate resistence form. Reduction should be accomplished during initial tooth preparation as it improves access and visibility for subsequent steps.

The goal is to achieve a final restoration with restored cusps having a minimal thickness of 2 mm for functional cusps and 1.5 mm for non-functional cusps, while developing an appropriate occlusal relationship.

When possible, opposing vertical walls should be formed to converge occlusally. Also, a facial or lingual groove may be extended arbitrarily to increase retention form. The pulpal and gingival walls should be relatively flat and perpendicular to the long axis of the tooth.

Final

After initial preparation, removal of any remaining infected carious dentin or removal of remaining old restorative material is usually necessary. A liner can be applied, if needed, and if used, should not extend closer than 1 mm to a slot or a pin.

Pins placed into prepared pinholes (or pin channels) provide auxiliary resistance and retention forms.

The depth of the pinhole varies from 1.3 - 2 mm depending on the diameter of the pin used. However, a general guideline for pinhole depth is 2 mm. The prepared pinhole is 0.0015 inch to 0.004 inch smaller than the diameter of the pin. These are for the most frequently used pin type-small self threading pins.

Friction locked and cemented pinsm although still available, are rarely used.

Another technique restores teeth with amalgam and cemented pins using threaded (or serrated) S.S. pins. Pinholes prepared are 0.001-0.002 inch larger than the diameter of the pin. The cementing medium may be any standard dental luting agent.

Technique using friction

Locked pin is also used in which the diameter of the pinhole is 0.001 inch smaller than the diameter of the pin. The pins are tapped into place, retained by the resiliency of the dentin and are 2-3 times more retentive than cemented pins.

Pin design

Four sizes of pins are available and for each size, several designs are available: standard; self shearing, 2 in 1, link series and link plus.

Pin-hole preparation

The roder drill (A twist drill) should be used. Drill is made of a high-speed tool steel that is swagged into an aluminium shank - (acts as a heat absirber; is color coded; matched with appropriate pin size. The optimal depth of pinhole into the dentim is 2 mm; so a depth-limiting drill should be used. Only when this type of drill prepares a hole on a flat surface that is perpendicular to the drill will it prepare the pinhole to the correct depth.

With the drill tip in its proper position andwith the handpiece rotating at very low speed (300-500 rpm), apply pressure to the drill and prepare the pinhole in one to two movements until until the depth-limiting portion of the drill is reached and remove the drill from the pinhole.

Although not usually recommended, a steady stream of air may be applied to be drill to dissipate heat.

Pin insertion

Two instruments for insertion of threaded pins are available:

1. Comentional latch - type contra - angle handpiece;
2. TMS hand wrenches.

The latch-type handpiece is recommended for insertion of link series and link plus; the hand wrench for standard pins.

L.Q.A.2 Classify pins ? What factors will you consider before using pins for amalgam restoration in a badly multilated tooth ? Describe the procedure of fixing a threaded pin?

Ans. The type of pins are:

- Self - threading pin,
- Friction - locked and,
- Cemented pins.

Four sizes of pins are available, each with a corresponding color coded drill.

Minuta - 0.015 inch (0.38 mm) (smallest)

Minikin - 0.019 inch (0.48 mm)

Minim - 0.024 inch (0.61 mm)

Regular - 0.031 inch (0.78 mm) (largest pin)

For each of 4 sizes of pins, several designs are available:

- Standard,
- Self-shearing,
- Two-in-one,
- Link series andlink plus.

Factors to be considered before using pins

The most frequently used pin type is the small self-threading pin. The pin-retained amalgam restoration using self-threading pins, the diameter of the prepared pinhole is 0.0015 inch to 0.004 inch smaller than the diameter of the pin. The threads engage the dentin as it is inserted, retaining the pin. The elasticity of the dentin permits insertion of a threaded pin into a hole of smaller diameter. Although the threads of self-threading pins do not engage the denin for their entire width, the self-threading pin is the most retentive of three types of pins.

The depth ofpinhole varies from 1.3-2 mm. A general guideline is 2 mm depth. Several types of self-threading pins are also available.

Pin insertion

A standard design pin is placed in the appropriate Wrench and slowly threaded clockwise into the pinhole until a definite resistance is felt when the pin reaches the bottom of the hole.

The pin should then be rotated one-quarter to one-half turn counter-clockwise to reduce the dentinal stress created by the end of the pin pressing dentin.

Once the pins are placed, evaluate their length. Any length of pin greater than 2 mm should be removed 2 mm of pin length into amalgam is optimal.

L.Q.A.3 Complex amalgam restorations

Ans. Complex posterior restorations are used to replace missing tooth structure of teeth that have fractured or are severely involved with caries or existing restorative material, These restorations usually involved the replacement of one or more missing cusps and often they utilize a bonding techniques.

Contra-indications

The complex amalgam restoration may be contra-indicated if the patient has significant occlusal problems or if the tooth cannot be properly treated with a direct restorationbecause of anatomic and / or functional considerations. The complex amalgam restoration may also be contra-indicated if the area to be restored is esthetically important.

Advantages

Conserves tooth structure: Preparation is usually more conservative that the preparation for an indirect restoration or a crown.

Appointment time: The complex restoration can be completed in one appointment. The cast restoration requires at least 2 appointments.

Resistance and retention form: May be significantly increased by the use of pins, slots and bonding.

Economics: Is a relatively inexpensive restorative procedure. Its the only alternative to extraction in severely carious teeth, when lost is a factor.

Disadvantages

Dentinal microfractures: Preparing pinholes and placing pins may create craze lines or fractures, as well as internal stresses in the dentin. Such craze lines and internal stress may have little or no clinical significance, but they may be important when minimal dentin is present.

Microleakage: In amalgam restorations using cavity varnish, microleakage around all types of pins has been demonstrated.

Decreased strength of amalgam: The tensile strength and horizontal strength of pin-retained amalgam restorations are significantly reduced.

Resistance form: Is more difficult to develop than when preparing a tooth for a cusp-capping only or a full crown. The complex amalgam restorations doesn't protect the tooth from fracture as well as an extracoronla restoration.

Penetration and perforation: Pin retention increases the risk of penetrating into the pulp or perforating the external tooth surface.

Tooth anatomy: Proper contours and occlusal contacts and / or anatomy are sometimes difficult to achieve wit h large complex restorations.

S.Q.A.1 Self-shearing pin

Ans. The link plus pins are self-shearing and are available as a single or two-in-one pin contained in a color coded plastic sleeve. This design has a sharper thread, a shoulder stop at 2 mm and a tapered tip to more readily fit the bottom of the pinhole as prepared by the twist drill. It also provides a 2.7 mm length of pin to extend out of the dentin, which usually needs to be shortened.

The self-shearing pin has a total length that varies according to the diameter of the pin. It also consists of a flattened head to engage the hand wrench or the appropriate handpiece huck for threading into the pinhole. When the pin approaches the bottom of the pinhole, the head of the pin shears off, leaving a length of pin extendin from the dentin.

The two-in-one pins is actually 2 pins in one, with each one being shorter than the standard pin. The 2-in-1 pin is approximately 9.5 mm in length and also has a flattened head to aid in its insertion.

When the pin reaches the bottom of the pinhole, it shears approximately in half, leaving a length a pin extending from the dentin with the other half remaining in the hand wrench or the handpiece chuck.

This second pin may be positioned in another pinhole and threaded to place in the same manner as the standard pin.

The minutea and minikin pins are available only in self-shearing and link (also self-shearing) design.

8 Restoration for Class–III, V & VI Cavity Preparation

L.Q.A.1 Compare and contrast cavities in anterior restoration ?

Ans. Class-III restorations are indicated for defects located on the proximal surface of anterior teeth that do not affect the incisal edge. Part of the facial or the lingual surfaces may also be involved in class III restoration.

Class-V are indicated to restore defects on the facial or lingual cervical one-third of any tooth.

Class-VI is used to restore the incisal edge of anterior teeth or the cusp tip regios of the posterior teeth.

Class-III amalgam restoration is used infrequently, its use has been supplanted by tooth colored restoration.

Class-V can be especially technically sensitive because of location, extent of caries and limited access and visibility.

Indications

Class III is usually reserved for distal surface of distal surface of maxillary and mandibular canine for esthetic reasons, amalgam is rarely indicated for the proximal surface of incisors and the mesial surface of canines.

Access for the tooth preparation is generally from the lingual approach, to conserve the enamel facial to the proximal contact.

Class V are also reserved for nonesthetic areas, where access and visibility are limited and where moisture control are limited and where moisture control is difficult and for areas that are deep gingivally, serves for a long time without failing.

Class-VI are in cases where attrition has remvoed the enamel to expose the underlying detin on those areas. The softer dentin wears off faster than surrounding enamel - "Cupped out" areas.

There may be sensitivity to hot and cold frequently and some patients are bothered by food impaction in the deeper depressions.

Amalgam may be selected especially (posterior class VI preparations) because of its wear resistance and longevity. Also indicated to restore hypoplastic pit occasionally found on cusp tips.

Advantages

Amalgam restorations are stronger than other class-III, V, and VI direct restorations. In addition are easier to place and may be less expensive, easier to finish and polish.

Disadvantage

Primary disadvantage is they are metallic and unesthetic.

Tooth preparation

Class-III

The outline form of class-III amalgam preparation on a canine is similar the conventional class-III composite. The amalgam uses a bur instead of a diamond and incorporates no enamel bevels. In addition, requires econdary retention features and a specific and uniform axial depth. A lingual devetail may be indicated if one existed previously of if additional retention is needed.

Class-V

Proper amalgam form for class-V amalgam preparations results in extending the cavosurface margins to sound tooth structure while maintaining a limited axial depth of 0.5 mm instead DEJ and 0.75 mm inside cementum. The outline form is primarily detemined by the location and size of the caries or old restorative material.

Class-VI

The area is entered with a small tapered fissure bur and extend to sufficient size to place the cavosurface margin on enamel that has sound dentin support. The preparation walls may need diverge occlusally to ensure a 90° cavosurface margin. A depth of 1.5 mm is sufficient for bulk and retention is created by small undercuts along the internal line angles.

L.Q.A.2 Discuss in detail the management of proximal caries in relation to upper anterior teeth ?

Ans.

Initial tooth preparation

- Bur size depends on the anticipated size of restoration. Usually a No. 2 bur is used. However, No. 1/2 or 1 should be used in small teeth or lesions.
- The bur is positioned so that entry cut will penetrate into lesion, which is usually gingival to contact area. The long axis of bur is positioned to be perpendicular to the lingual surface but directed at a mesial angle close to the adjacent tooth.

  Penetration should be at a limited initial axial depth 0.5 - 0.6 mm inside DEJ or at a 0.75-0.8 mm when gingival margin is in cementum.

  Infected dentin that is deeper that this initial axial depth is removed later during final tooth preparation.
- For smal l lesion, facial margin is extended 0.2-0.3 mm into facial embrasure with a curved outline from incisal to gingival margin.

  The lingual outline blends with the incisal and gingival margins in a smooth curve, creating a preparation with little or no lingual wall.
- The cavosurface angle should be 90° at all margins. The facial, incisal and gingival margins should meet axial wall at approx. right angles.
- The initial axial wall depth may be in sound dentin, in infected dentin or in existing restorative material.
- When preparing a gingival wall that is near either the level of rubber dam or apical to it, a wedge should be used - triangular than round for a deep gingival margin.

- The initial tooth preparation is completed by using a No. 1/2 bur. This bur smoothes any roughened, undermined enamel produced at the gingival and facial cavosurface margins.

Final tooth preparation

May involve removing any removing any remaining infected dentin, protecting the pulp, developing secondary resistance and retention forms, finishing external walls and the final procedures of cleaning, inspecting and desensitizing or bonding.

A small round revolving bur or appropriate spoon excavators or both are used to remove remaining infected carious dentin.

Resistance form is provided by:

- Cavosurface and amalgam margins of 90°.
- Enamel walls supported by sound dentin.
- Sufficient bulk of amalgam and
- No sharp preparation initial angles.

The box like preparation form provides primary retention form.

Secondary form is by a gingival groove, an incisal cone and sometimes, a lingual donetail.

After preparation of retention forms, remove any unsupported enamel, smooth enamel walls and margins and refine the cavosurface angles where indicated. If gingival margin is in enamel, a slight bevel of 20° is necessary.

The completed tooth preparation is carefully cleaned and inspected. Desensitizers or bonding agents are used as a part of the final preparation and restorative stages.

L.Q.A.3 What are the advantages of composite resin restoration materials? Describe the procedure for acid-etching & restoring a cavity with composite resin?

Ans. The term composite material may be defined as a compound of two or more distinctly different materials with properties that are superior or intermediate to those of the individual constituents.

Composite resin is basically a resin which has been strengthened by adding silica particles.

Advantages

- Restoration of anterior & posterior teeth (directly or as inlays)
- To veneer metal crowns & bridges.
- To build up cores
- Cementation of orthodontic brackets, Maryland bridges & ceramic crowns, inlays, onlays & laminates
- Pit & fissure sealants
- Esthetics laminates
- Repair of chipped porcelain restorations.

Acid etching

The acid etch technique is one of the most effective ways of improving the bond & marginal seal between resin & enamel.

It forms the basis for many other dental procedures like resin-bonded metal retainers porcelain laminate veneers & orthodontic brackets

Mode of action

- It creates microporosities by discrete etching of the enamel i.e. by selective dissolution of enamel rodcenters or peripheries or both.
- It increases the surface area.
- Etched enamel has a high surface energy allowing resin to wet the tooth surface better & penetrate into the microporosities. When polymerized it forms *"resin tags"* which form a mechanical bond to the enamel.

Acid used - 37 % Phosphoric acid

- Supplied as a colored gel.
- Brushes are used to apply or the acid is supplied in a syringe and can be dispensed onto the enamel

Procedure

- Clean & polish tooth with pumice

- Acid is then applied onto the enamel
- Initially was 60 secs, but now recommended - 15 secs.
- Rinse thoroughly with a stream of water for 15 secs.
- Thoroughly dry enamel
- Enamel should have a white frosted appearance
- Keep surface clean & dry & place resin
- Contamination with saliva (or blood) can prevent effective tag formation & severely reduce the bond strength.

L.Q.A.4 Describe the procedure of restoring abrasive defect (CLASS-V restoration) ?

Ans. Class-V modified tooth preparations are used to restore abraded or eroded cervical areas. Abrasion, in the form of a notch, often V-shaped, is a loss or wearing away of tooth structure due to mechanical forces, such as strenuous toothbrushing with a hard bristle toothbrush or abrasive toothpaste.

Tooth preparation for a class-V abrasion area usually requires only roughening of the internal walls with a diamond instrument; beveling or flaring all enamel margins; & sometimes, placing a retention groove in non-enamel areas. If necessary, prepare the root-surface cavosurface margins to approximately 90°. Often the inherent form of abraded lesion will result in no need for further preparation of root-surface cavosurface margins. Retention groove may not be needed, but, greater restoration retention may be provided when the retention groove is utilized.

The restoration of an abrasion lesion needs proper insertion technique for a *light-cured material.* Following etching & priming steps for enamel & dentin, a thin layer of bonding adhesive is placed & cured. Then the composite is inserted incrementally with a hand instrument or syringe. The deep preparations having retentive undercuts need to be filled atleast in 2 increments. First, a small amount of material is inserted in the retentive undercuts and cured. Second, the outer portion of the preparation is filled & the material shaped as close to the final contour shaped as possible. An explorer or blade of a composite instrument is used to remove excess material from cervical margin & obtaining the final contour. Then the light source is applied for polymerization. The restoration requires very little finishing.

Because of the limited strength & wear resistance, *glass ionomers* are indicated for low stress areas where caries activity potential is of a significant concern. Hence its use is recommended for root-surface caries in class V locations. Notched cervical defects of abrasion origin also are well-suited for restorations with GIC, if esthetics is not a concern. The tooth preparations are the same as that for composite restorations.

L.Q.A.5 What are the clinical indications for GIC? What do you understand by 'SANDWICH TECHNIQUE'. Write in detail the restoration of a class V erosion lesion in a posterior tooth ?

Ans. **Indications**

- Anterior esthetic restorative material for class III cavities
- For eroded areas & class V restorations
- As a luting agent
- As liners & bases
- For core build up
- To a limited extent as pit & fissure sealants.

Sandwich technique

Composite does not bond adequately to dentin, therefore during polymerization, a gap may result if the cavity margin is situated in dentin.

The bond to dentin can be improved by placing a GIC liner between the composite restoration & dentin.

The GI bonds to the dentin through chemical adhesion whereas the resin bonds mechanically to porosities & crazing present on the surface of the GI liner.

The GI can also be etched with the help of phosphoric acid to improve retention. It also provides an anticariogenic effect due to its fluoride release.

This types of procedure is often referred to as SANDWICH TECHNIQUE.

Indications

- Lesions where one or more margins are in dentin e.g. Cervical lesions.
- Class-II composite restorations.

Procedure

- Dentin is conditioned.
- A thin layer of GIC is placed such that its exposed at the margins to achieve fluoride release.
- Phosphoric acid is used to etch the enamel portion (GIC surface can also be etched.)
- After adequate drying, a bond agent is applied.
- Composite resin then inserted in the usual manner.

L.Q.A.6 Mention various anterior restoration materials & describe a technique of restoring class-III cavity while using any 1 of them ?

Ans. The anterior restorations are reasons of esthetic concern. Many esthetic restorative materials are available, also called as tooth-colored restoration. These are:

- Silicate cement.
- Acrylic resin.

Composite

- Conventional composite.
- Microfill composites.
- Hybrid composites.
- Flowable composites.
- Packable composites.

Glass ionomer

- Conventional glass ionomers.
- Resin-modified glass ionomers.
- Compomers (polyacid-modified composites).

Techniques

Clinical technique for direct class-III composite restorations:

Initial clinical procedures

Anesthesia may be necessary for patient comfort & if used, will decrease salivary flow.

Occlusal assessments should be made to help in properly adjusting the restoration's function & in determining the tooth preparation design.

The shade must be selected before the tooth dehydrates & experiences concomitant lightening. The area must be isolated to permit effective bonding. If the restoration will be large, prewedging the area will assist in reestablishment of proximal contact.

Tooth preparation

Class-III preparations by definition, are located on the proximal surfaces of anterior teeth. Such locations are predominant site for composites for esthetics & are retained mainly due to the micro-mechanical bond from etching & bonding, so no additional retention form necessary.

Sometimes groove or cove may be needed for extensions onto the root surface or ones that are very large.

The lingual approach for restoration is preferred for esthetic reasons.

Beveled conventional class-III

The beveled conventional tooth preparation for composite restorations is indicated primarily for replacing an existing defective restoration in the crown portion of the tooth. However it may also be used when restoring a large carious lesion for which the need for increased retention &/or resistance is anticipated. The tooth preparation takes shape of the existing restoration along with any extensions necessary to include recurrent caries, friable tooth structure, or defects. The beveled conventional preparation is characterized by external walls that are perpendicular to the enamel surface, with the enamel margin beveled. The axial line angles may or may not be of uniform pulpal depth, varying as the thickness of the enamel portion of the external walls varies. If part of the root surface is to be restored too, a combination of conventional type in the root portion & a beveled conventional type in the crown portion.

Lingual access

A round carbide bur (no. ½, 1, or 2) or diamond stone, the size depending on the extent of the caries or defective restoration, to prepare the outline form. Before contacting the tooth, the cutting instrument is positioned for entry & rotated at very high speed using air-water spray. The point of entry is within the inciso-gingival dimension of the carious lesion or defective restoration & as close to the adjacent tooth as possible without contacting it. The cutting instrument is directed perpendicular to the enamel surface, but at an angle that places the neck portion of the bur as far into the embrasure as possible; light pressure & intermittent cutting is used to gain access into the lesion. The same instrument may be used to enlarge the opening sufficiently to allow for the caries removal, completion of the preparation & insertion of the restorative material.

The external walls are extended to sound tooth structure during preparation of the outline form, to the initial limited prescribed depth. This extension is dictated by the extent of caries &/or old restorative material on these walls. The axial wall depth is limited to 0.2mm inside the DEJ, which means it will be approx. 0.75 to 1.25 mm deep. The axial wall will be outwardly convex, following normal external tooth contour & the DEJ, both insicogingivally & faciolingually. Usually the axial line angles should be at an initial depth of 0.2mm into dentin. The axial depth should not be exceeded at this stage, any remaining infected dentin, or old defective restorative material on the axial wall will be removed during final preparation.

The enamel walls are prepared perpendicular to the external tooth surface. The gingival floor & lingual wall usually finished with the same round cutting instrument.

Once the outline form & axial wall depth are established, the initial preparation is completed. All remaining infected dentin is removed using round burs or small excavators, or both. Very friable enamel is removed. Calcium hydroxide liner applied if indicated.

If retention features are indicated, its prepared along the gingivoaxial line angle & sometimes the incisoaxial line angle with a no. ¼ bur.

Class-III beveled conventional tooth preparations are prepared are prepared as conventional preparations with addition of a cavosur face bevel or flare of the enamel rather a butt joint margin. Its best prepared by a flame-shaped or round diamond instrument, resulting in an angle approx. 45° to the external tooth surface. A bevel width of 0.25 to 0.5 mm is considered sufficient.

For moderate & large class-III beveled conventional preparations, all accessible enamel margins usually are beveled, with the exception of the gingival margin.

Clean the preparation of any visible debris & inspect for final approval.

Restoration technique

Etching, priming & placing adhesives: First the proximal surface of the adjacent unprepared tooth is protected from inadvertent etching by placing a polyster strip. Then a gel etchant is applied to all of the prepared tooth structure, approx. 0.5 mm beyond the preparation margins onto the adjacent tooth. The etchant is left undisturbed for 15 to 30 secs. The area is then washed. The dentin surface should remain moist, a glistening appearance.

The primer is applied to all of the prepared tooth structure with a microbrush or other applicator tip. If dry spots remain, an additional coat or coats of primer are indicated.

If the bonding system does not combine the primer & adhesive, the bonding adhesive is applied next. Another microbrush or applicator tip is used. Once applied, the adhesive is polymerized with the curing light as directed.

Matrix application: a matrix is a device that is applied to a prepared tooth before the insertion of the restorative material. It aids in placing, confining, & contouring the composite material, and also aid in isolating the preparation.

A properly contoured polyster strip matrix is used for most class III & IV preparations. A wedge is needed at the gingival margin when all of the proximal contact is involved. An end of a round wooden toothpick approx. 3/8 inch long usually is an excellent wedge.

Inserting & curing composite

Placed in two stages – first, a bonding adhesive applied (if not applied earlier) & then composite material inserted. There are two types:

self-cured & light cured. Either is preferred and dispensed, inserted in the cavity & cured

S.Q.A.1 Mention various anterior restorative materials

Ans.

Various anterior restorative materials

For most anterior restorations, esthetic material such as composite is indicated almost always.

- Microfill composites are indicated promarily for small class III, class V and partial veneer restorations.
- Glass ionomer may be the material of choice for restoring rootsurface caries in high caries activity and where esthetics is not as critical.
- A veneer is a layer of tooth-colored material that is applied to a tooth to restore localized or generalized defects and intrinsic discoloration. Typically, veneers are made of chair-side composite, processed composite, procelain or pressed ceramic material.

Amalgam restorations may be indicated in distal surface of maxillary and mandibular canines. May also be used for class V and Vi restorative procedures. Its used in cases where in esthetics is not a primary concern.

9 Cast Metal Restorations for Class-II Restorations

L.Q.A.1 What is an inlay? How will you prepare a class-II cavity on maxillary first molar for cast gold restorations?

Ans. The class II inlay involves the occlusal & proximal surfaces of a posterior tooth & may cap one or more, but not all of the cusps. The procedure requires 2 appointments: the first for preparing the tooth & making an impression & the second for delivering the restoration to the patient. The fabrication process is referred to as an indirect procedure because the casting is made on a replica of the prepared tooth in a dental laboratory.

When a maxillary first molar is to be restored, consideration should be given to preserving the oblique ridge if it is strong & unaffected, especially if only one proximal surface is carious. A small distal cavitated, carious lesion is described here:

Initial preparation

Carbide burs are used to develop the vertical internal walls of the preparation. The side and end surfaces of the bur should be straight to aid in the development of uniformly tapered walls & smooth pulpal & gingival walls. Suggested burs are the No.271 & the No.169L. The marginal bevels are placed with a slender, fine-grit, flame shaped diamond instrument, such as the No.8862.

Throughout the preparation for a cast inlay, the cutting instruments used to develop the vertical walls are oriented to a single 'draw' path, usually the long axis of the tooth crown,so that the completed preparation will have draft (no undercut).

The gingival to occlusal divergence may range from 2-5 degrees per wall from the line of draw.

Occlusal step

With the No. 271 carbide bur held parallel to the long axis of the tooth crown, enter the fossa or pit closest to the involved marginal ridge,using a punch cut to a depth of 1.5 mm to establish the depth of the pulpal wall. The bur should be rotating at high speed before application to the tooth & should not stop rotating until it is removed. A general rule is to maintain the long axis of the bur parallel to the long axis of the tooth crown at all times. The cutting should be done at high speeds with a properly directed air-water spray to provide the necessary cooling & cleansing effects.

Maintaining the 1.5 mm initial depth & the same bur orientation, extend the preparation outline mesially along the central groove/fissure to include mesial fossa/pit. Extend to include faulty facial and lingual fissures radiating from the mesial pit. The final extension of these fissures can be accomplished with the slender No. 169L carbide bur.

Tooth structure & strength can be further conserved by

1. Enameloplasty of the fissure ends should be employed when possible &
2. The marginal bevel of the final preparation is used to include the terminal ends of these fissures in the outline form.

The facial & lingual extensions in the mesial pit region should provide the desired dovetail retention form, which resists distal displacement of the inlay.

Continuing at the initial depth, the oclusal step is extended distally into the distal marginal ridge sufficiently to expose the junction of the proximal enamel & the dentin. While extending distally, progressively the preparation is widened to the desired facio-lingual width in anticipation for the proximal box preparation. This increased faciolingual width enables the facial and lingual walls of the box to project perpendicularly to the proximal surface that will clear the adjacent tooth by 0.2 to 0.5 mm. The facial & lingual walls of the occlusal step should go around the cusps in curves & the prepared isthmus in the transverse ridge ideally should be only slightly wider than the bur, thus conserving dentinal protection for the pulp & maintaining strength of the cusps.

Proximal box

Continuing with No. 271 carbide bur, isolate the distal enamel by cutting a proximal ditch. Slight pressure toward enamel is necessary to avoid the bur from cutting only dentin. Ideal extension gingivally of a minimal, cavitated lesion will eliminate caries on the gingival floor & provide 0.5 mm clearance of the unbeveled gingival margin with the adjacent tooth.

When preparing the proximal portion of the preparation, maintain the side of the bur at the specified axial wall depth regardless of whether it is in dentin, caries, old restorative material, or air.

Then with the No.271 carbide bur, make 2 cuts, one at the facial limit of the proximal ditch and the other at the lingual limit, extending from the ditch perpendicularly towards the enamel surface. Extend these cuts until the bur is nearly through the marginal ridge enamel.

Planing the distofacial, distolingual & gingival walls by hand instruments to remove all undermined enamel may be indicated. Depending on access, use a No.15 (width) straight chisel, biangle chisel or enamel hatchet. Usually, experienced operator don't use chisels but use the narrow, flame shaped, fine-grit diamond instrument.

Shallow (0.3 mm deep) retention grooves may be cut in the facioaxial & linguoaxial line angles with the No.169L carbide bur. These are indicated when the tooth is short.

Final preparation

Removal of infected carious dentin & pulp protection

With slowly revolving bur or spoon excavator, is used to remove the carious infected dentin. If the excavation closely approaches the pulp or if a direct pulp cap is indicated, a lining of calcium hydroxide to cover & protect any possible near or actual exposure & also extend over a major portion of the excavated dentin surface.

Preparation of bevels & flares

The slender, flame shaped, fine-grit diamond instrument is used to bevel the occlusal & gingival margins & to apply the secondary flare on the distolingual & distofacial walls. This should result in 30-40 degree marginal metal on the inlay. The flame shaped diamond instrument, rotating at high speed, is used to prepare the lingual secondary flare & is approached from the lingual embrasure, moving the instrument mesiofacially. On comparing the direction of the distolingual wall & the position of the distolingual margin before & after this extension, its seen that the distolingual wall extends from the linguoaxial line angle into the lingual embrasure in 2 planes: the first is termed the lingual primary flare; the second is the lingual secondary flare. During this secondary flare, the long axis of the instrument is held nearly parallel to the line of draw, with only a slight tilting mesially & lingually for assurance of draft & the direction of translation of the instrument is that which results in a marginal metal angle of 40 degrees.

Bevel the gingival margin by moving the instrument facially along the gingival margin, to create a 30 degree marginal metal by slightly tilting the instrument mesially. The gingival bevel must be 0.5-1mm wide & should blend with the lingual secondary flare.

The flame-shaped, fine grit diamond instrument is also used for occlusal bevels.the width of the cavosurface bevel on the occlusal margin should be approx. one fourth the depth of the respective wall. The resulting occlusal marginal metal of the inlay should be 40-degree metal,thus he occlusal marginal enamel is 140-degree enamel.

The diamond instrument also is used to lightly bevel the axiopulpal line angle.

Thus the desirable metal angle margins of inlay is 40-degrees, except the gingival margins where it should be 30 degrees.

L.Q.A.2 **Discuss modifications of the different cavity designs for class II cavities for cast gold restorations?**

Ans.

Mesioocclusodistal prepation

If the marginal ridge is severly weakened because of excessive extension, the preparation outline often should be altered to include the proximal surface. E.g. A DO should be extended into an MOD preparation.

For esthetics

For esthetic reasons, minimal flare is desired for the mesiofacial proximal wall in maxillary premolars & 1st molars. Its extended facially in such a way that the margin is barely visible from facial viewing position. The secondary flare in such cases is omitted.

Facial or lingual surface groove extensions

The extension of the preparation is done to include the faulty fissures. This may also provide as improved retention forms. These must be beveled. Just like the gingival margin.

Preparation for abutment teeth & extension gingivally to include root-surface lesions

Extending the facial, lingual & gingival margins may be indicated on the proximal surfaces of the abutments for removable partial dentures to increase the surface area for development of guiding planes. In addition, the occlusal outline form must be wide enough facio-lingually to accommodate any contemplated rest preparation(s) without involving the margins of the restoration. These are accomplishes by increasing the width of the bevels.

When further gingival extension is indicated to include a root lesion on the proximal surface: the gingival extension is accomplished primarily by lengthening the gingival bevel, especially when preparing a tooth that has a longer clinical crown than normal as a result of gingival recession. It is necessary to only slightly extend he gingival floor & although the axial wall consequently must be moved pulpally, it should be minimal.

Maxillary 1st molar with unaffected, strong oblique ridge: mq 1.

If a distal surface lesion appears subsequently to insertion of a MO restoration, the tooth may be prepared for a distoocclusolingual inlay. This inlay caps the distolingual cusp & is preferable to a DO restoration.

Fissures in the facial & lingual cusp ridges or marginal ridges

In the preparation of class-II for inlays, facial & lingual occlusal fissures may extend nearly to, or through, the respective facial & lingual cusp ridges, but not onto the facial or lingual surface. Proper outline form dictates that the preparation margin should not cross such fissures, but should be extended to include them.

L.Q.A.3 Mention the various factors that contribute for the retention of cast restorations. Describe the procedure of taking direct wax pattern after cavity preparation is completed.

Ans. Various factors for retention of cast restorations

Cast metal intracoronal restorations rely primarily on almost parallel vertical (longitudinal) walls to provide retention of the casting in the tooth.

During initial tooth preparation, the preparation walls must be designed not only to provide for draw or draft (in order for the casting to be placed in the tooth), but also to provide for an appropriate small angle of divergence (2 to 5 degrees per wall) from the line of draw that will enhance retention form. The degree of divergence needed primarily depends on the length of the prepared walls: the greater the vertical height of the walls, the more divergence is permitted & recommended, but within the range described.

In inlay or onlay preparations for cast metal restorations, the opposing vertical walls diverge outwardly by only a few degrees to each other & to a draw path that is usually perpendicular to the floor of the preparation. Having sufficient length of these almost parallel walls allow enough frictional resistance & mechanical locking of the luting agent into minute irregularities of both the casting & the preparation walls to counteract the pull of sticky foods. Close parallelism of prepared vertical walls is a principal retention form for cast metal restorations, another being the use of luting agent that bonds to tooth stucture.

Direct wax pattern procedure

The first procedure in the casting of an inlay or crown for the lost-wax process is the preparation of a wax pattern. The cavity is prepared in the tooth & the pattern is carved, either directly in the tooth or on a die that is a reproduction of the tooth & the prepared cavity. If the pattern is made within the tooth, it is said to be prepared by the direct technique.

Manipulation

Dry heat is generally preferred to the use of water-bath. When stick wax is softened over flame, care should be taken not to overheat it. It should be twirled until it becomes shiny & then removed from the flame. The process is repeated until the wax is warm throughout. It is then kneaded together & shaped to the prepared cavity. Type I wax has enough plasticity in a temperature range safely tolerated by the pulp. Pressure should be applied by the finger or by the patient biting on the wax. It is cooled gradually at mouth temperature, not by cold water.

Care should be exercised in removing the pattern. It should be hooked with an explorer point & rotated out of the cavity. A MOD pattern can best be removed by luting a staple so that each prong is fastened above a corresponding step portion. It can then be removed with dental floss looped through the staple & withdrawn in a direction parallel to the axial walls & with minimum distortion. After removal, touching with fingers should be avoided as much as possible to prevent any temperature changes. The pattern should be immediately invested after removal from the mouth.

L.Q.A.4 What are the different cast restorations on molars fabricated? Briefly give their indications? Give an account of defects on fabrication.

Ans. The cast metal restoration is versatile & is especially applicable to class-II onlay preparations.

The class-II inlay involves the occlusal & proximal surfaces of a posterior tooth & may cap one or more, but not all cusps. The class-II onlay involves the proximal surfaces of a posterior tooth & caps all of the cusps.

INDICATIONS

Large restorations

The cast metal inlay is an alternative to amalgam or composite when the higher strength of a casting alloy is needed or when the superior control of contours or contacts that the indirect procedure provides is desired. The cast metal onlay is often an excellent alternative to a crown for teeth that have been greatly weakened by caries or large, failing restoration(s), but the facial & lingual tooth surfaces are relatively unaffected by disease or injury. When proximal surface caries is extensive, favorable consideration should be given to the cast inlay or onlay. The indirect procedure used to develop the cast restoration allows more control of contours & contacts.

Endodontically treated tooth

A molar or premolar with endodontic treatment can be restored with a cast metal onlay providing the onlay has been thoughtfully designed to strengthen the remaining tooth.

Teeth at risk for fracture

Fracture lines in enamel & dentin, especially in teeth having extensive restorations, should be recognized as cleavage planes for possible future fracture of tooth. Restoring these teeth with a restoration that braces the tooth against fracture injury may sometimes be warranted. Such restorations are cast onlays (with skirting) & crowns.

Dental rehabilitation with cast metal alloys

When cast metal restorations have been used to restore adjacent or opposing teeth, the continued use of same material may be considered to eliminate electrical or corrosive activity that sometimes occurs between dissimilar metals in mouth, particularly when they contact each other.

Diastema closure & occlusal plane correction

Often a cast inlay or onlay is indicated when extension of the mesiodistal dimension of the tooth is necessary to form a contact with an adjacent tooth. Cast onlays also can be used to correct the occlusal plane of a slightly tilted tooth.

Removable prosthodontic abutment

Teeth that are to serve as abutments for a removable partial denture can be restored with a cast metal restoration.

Major advantages

- The superior physical properties of the cast metal alloy allow it to better withstand the forces imparted by the partial denture, &
- The rest seats, guiding planes, & other aspects of contour relating to partial denture are better controlled when the indirect technique is used.

DEFECTS

Occur when proper procedure is not followed. The castings then are not fit or may have poor esthetic & mechanical properties.

Classification

- Distortion
- Surface roughness
- Porosity
- Incomplete casting
- Sulphur compounds due to breakdown of the investment when the ring is overheated.

Distortion: Due to distortion of wax patten

- When investment hardens or due to hygroscopic & setting expansion.
- During manipulation due to release of stresses.

Surface roughness: Due to:

- Air bubbles in wax pattern
- Too rapid heating causing fins
- Higher w/p ratio
- Prolonged heating causing disintegration of mould cavity
- Overheating of gold alloy – disintegrates the investment
- Too high or too low casting pressure
- Proportion of quartz & binder affects the surface texture. Coarse silica- coarse casting.
- Foreign body inclusions show sharp well defined deficiencies.

Porosity: May be internal or external.

External: Discoloration.

Internal: Weakens the restoration.

Incomplete casting:

- Insufficient alloy
- Alloy unable to enter thin parts of mould.
- Mould not heated to casting temperature

- Premature solidification of alloy
- Sprues blocked with foreign bodies
- Back pressure due to gases in mould cavity
- Low casting pressure.
- Alloy not sufficiently molten or fluid.

L.Q.A.6 What precautions will you take to prevent the defects in cast gold restoration?

Ans.

Precautions to prevent defects in cast gold restorations are

Distortion: Avoid by –

- Manipulation of wax at high temperature
- Investing pattern within one hour aften finishing
- If storage necessary, store in refrigerator

Surface roughness

- ***Air bubbles:*** Avoid by –
  - Proper mixing of investment
  - Vibration of mix or by vacuum investing
  - Application of wetting agent
- ***Fins:*** Avoided by heating the ring gradually to 700°C (in atleast 1 hr)
- ***W/P ratio:*** Use correct ratio
- Complete the casting as soon as the ring is heated and ready to avoid prolonged heating.
- Use 15 lbs / sq. inch of air pressure or 3–4 turns of centrifugal casting machine

Porosity

- ***To avoid lolalized shrinkage porosity:***
  - Use sprue of correct thickness
  - Attach sprue to thickest portion of wax pattern

  - Flaring the sprue to the point of attachment or placing a reservoir close to wax pattern.
- Suck back porosity is avoided by reducing the temperature difference between the mould & the molten alloy.
- ***Back pressure porosity avoided by:***
  - Using adequate casting force
  - Use investment of adequate porosity.
  - Place pattern not more than 6-8 mm away from the end of the ring
  - Providing vents in large casting.
- Gas blow holes. Avoided by doing the burnout with the sprue hole facing downwards.

Contamination: avoided by:

- Not overheating alloy
- Use reducing zone of the flame
- Use flux.

S.Q.A.1 Mention the precautions to be taken in avoiding distortion of the direct wax pattern in a MOD cavity in tooth no. 26 after cavity preparation is complete?

Ans.

Precautions

Distortion is probably the most serious problem experienced when forming & removing the pattern from mouth or die. It results from thermal changes & the release of stresses that arise from contraction on cooling, occluded air, change of shape during molding, carving, removal, & time & temperature during storage.

- Use of water-bath for manipulation results in inclusion of water droplets that distorts the pattern during thermal changes. Dry heat is preferred.
- Pressure should be applied by the finger or by the patient biting on the wax.

- It should be cooled gradually at mouth temparature, not by cold water.
- Care should be taken to remove the pattern from the cavity with minimum distortion.
- After removal touching with fingers should be avoided to prevent any temperature changes.to avoid delayed distortion, the pattern must be invested immediately after removal. Once the investment hardens, there will be no more distortion.

S.Q.A.2 Give indication of gold inlay ?

Ans. **Indication**- Indications of gold inlay according to type:

Type-I soft: Small inlays class-III & class-V cavities – when not subjected to great stress they are easily burnished.

Type-II medium: Inlays subject to moderate stress, thick ¾ crowns, abutments, pontics, full crowns & sometimes soft saddles.

Type-III hard: Inlays crowns & bridges, situations where there may be great stresses involved they usually can be age hardened.

Type-IV extra hard: Inlays subjected to very high stresses, partial denture framework & long span bridges. They can be age hardened.

S.Q.A.3 Disadvantages of cast restorations ?

Ans.

Number of appointments and higher chair time: The cast inlay requires atleast 2 appointments & much more time than a direct restoration, such as amalgam or composite.

Temporary: Patients must have temporary restorations between the preparation & delivery appointment. Temporaries occasionally loosen & or break, requiring additional visits.

Cost: The cost of material, laboratory bills & the time involved make indirect restorations more expensive than direct restorations.

Technique sensitive: Every step requires diligence & attention to detail. Errors at any part of the long, multistep process tends to be compounded, resulting in a less than optimal restoration.

Splitting forces: Small inlays may produce a wedging effect on facial &/ or lingual tooth structure, & thereby increase the potential for splitting the tooth.

S.Q.A.4 Casting shrinkage ?

Ans. Solidification defects (shrinkage) may cause:

- Localized shrinkage porosity
- Suck back porosity irregular in shape
- Microporosity

Localized shrinkage porosity

Is generally Caused by incomplete feeding of molten metal during solidification.

These are large irregular voids usually found near the spruce – casting function.

It occurs when the cooling sequence is incorrect & the spruce freezes before the rest of the casting.

During a correct cooling sequence, the spurce should freeze last. This allowes more molten metal to flow into the mould to compensate for the shrinkage of the casting as it solidifies.

It the spruce solidifies before rest of the casting no more molten metal can be supplied from the spruce.

The subsequent shrinkage produces voids or pits known as shrinkspot porosity.

Suck-Back porosity

- Is a variation of shrink spot porosity
- This is an external void usually seen in the inside of a crown opposite the spruce. A hot spot is created by the hot metal impinging on the mould wall near the spruce.
- The hot spot causes this region to freeze last. Since the spruce has already solidified, no more molten material is available & the resultant shrinkage causes.

Micro-porosity

Fine irregular voids within the lasting seen when casting freezes too rapidly (low temperature)

S.Q.A.5 Significance of reservoir ?

Ans. A reservoir should be added to a sprucing network to present localized shrinkage porosity.

A reservoir is positioned between the pattern & the crucible former.

When the molten alloy fills the heated casting ring the pattern area should solidity first & the reservoir last.

Because of its large mass of alloy & position in the heat center of the ring, the reservoir remains molten to furnish liquid alloy into the mold as it solidifies.

The resutting solidification shrinkage. Occurs in the reservoir bar & not in the restoration (assuming that the reservoir in larger in volume than the pattern & the sprue former attached were in proper position & of correct guage.)

S.Q.A.6 Hygroscopic expansion ?

Ans. When gypsum products are allowed to set in contact with water the amount of expansion exhibited is greater than the normal setting expansion the increased amount of expansion is because, water helps outward growth of crystals. This is known as HYGROSCOPIC SETTING EXPANSION. The investment should be immersed in water before initial set is complete.

ADA sp. No 2 for type II investment requires a minimal 1.2% & max 2.2% expension.

Factors affecting

Composition: Finer the particle size of silica greater SE

1. a - Hemihydcate produces a greater expansion than b.
2. Higher the silica greater the expansion.

W:P ratio: Higher W:P ratio, less HSE.

Temperature: Higher temperature greater expansion,

Effect of time of immersion: Before initial set, greater expansion.

Spatulation: Shorter the mixing time, less HSE,

Effect of shelf life: Older material less expansion.

Confinement: Of the the investment within the walls of the container or the wax pattern reduces HSE.

Effect of amount of added water: More water during setting expansion more expansion.

S.Q.A.7 Phosphate bonded investment material

Ans. Uses - For casting high fusing alloys.

Supplied as – Powder in packets with special liquid.

Composition

Powder

- Ammonium diacid phosphate
- It gives strength at room temperature
- It soluble in water & provides phosphate ions.
- Reacts with silica at high temperature to increase strength at casting temperatures.
- Silica – refractory
- Magnesium oxide – Reacts with phosphate ions.

Liquid: Is a form of silica sol in water (gives higher thermal expansion).

Setting reactions

At room temperature ammonium diacid phosphate reacts with magnesium oxide to give the investment green strength or room temperature strength.

$$NH_4H_2PO_4 + MgO + 5H_2O \rightarrow NH_4Mg\ (PO_4) + H_2O + Heat$$

Manipulation

The powder is mixed with a measured amount of liquid using a bowl & spatula.

Hand mixing or mechanical mixing under vacuum can be done.

The mixed material is vibrated into the casting ring or agar mould (RPD framework).

S.Q.A.8 Sprue

Ans. Is the channel in a refractory investment mold through which molten metal flows. A spruce former is created & attached to the wax pattern & it is surrounded with investment.

After the investment hardens, the spruce former is removed. The wax is also eliminated by boiling in water or by burning it but in an oven process called 'Burnout'.

The molten metal is then forced into the mold cavity left by the wax, through the spruce or ingate created by the spruce former.

This spruce helps compensate for alloy shrinkage during solidification by creating a reservoirs (which solidifies last & prevent localized shrinkages).

S.Q.A.9 Pressure casting ?

Ans. Too high a pressure during casting can produce a rough surface on the casting. A guage pressure of 0.10 to 0.14 Mpa in an air pressure casting machine or three to four turns of the spring in an average type of centrifugal casting machine is sufficient for a small casting.

10

Direct Gold Restorations

L.Q.A.1 What are the types of direct gold filling? Describe compaction technique & its use in dentistry ? How is a gold foil restoration finished ?

Ans.

Direct golds

Are those restorative materials that are manufactured for compaction directly into prepared cavities. Two types of direct golds are manufactured.

For dental use

Gold foil & powdered gold; they differ in their mettalurgic structure.

There are several physical types of direct-filling golds produced. All are compatible, in that, they are inserted into tooth preparations under force & compacted or condensed into preparation line & point angle & against preparation walls.

Gold foil

Manufactured by beating pure gold into thin sheets. The gold foil is cut into 4 × 4 inch sheets & sold in books of sheets, separated by pages of thin paper. The books contain 1/10th or 1/20th oz of gold. The sheets of foil that weigh 4gr each are termed no. 4 foil; the sheets weighing 3gr are termed no.3 foil & those weighing 2gr are no.2 foil. These sheets are rolled into cylinders or pellets before insertion in the tooth. The pellets are generally rolled from 1/32, 1/43, 1/64, or 1/128 inch sections cut from a no. 4 sheet of foil. Cylinders of foil maybe rolled from segments of a sheet.

Powdered gold

Made by combination of chemical precipitation & atomization, with an average particle size of 15mm. The atomized particles are mixed together in wax, cut into pieces, & wrapped in no.4 or no.3 foil. Several sizes of these pellets are available. This product is marketed as Williams E-Z Gold.

Compaction technique

Direct filling golds must be compacted during insertion into tooth preparations. With the exception of E-Z Gold, the compaction takes the form of malleting forces that are delivered either by a hand mallet used by the assistant or by an Electro-Mallet or a pneumatic mallet. E-Z Gold, because of its powdered form, maybe compacted by heavy hand pressure delivered in a motion with a specially designed hand condensers.

Preferred technique is use of hand mallet to deliver blows to a condenser; allows great control of malleting forces & allows for rapid change in condenser nibs, or tips, when multitude of condensers is required.

Two fundamental principles involved in compaction of cohesive gold are to:

- Weld the gold into a cohesive mass and
- Wedge as much gold as possible into the tooth preparation.

Welding takes place primarily as a result of the coherence of a noble metal to itself.

Wedging results from careful compacting technique

Gold foil compacts readily because of its thin form & produces a mass of linear channels of microporosity. Because the thin folds of the gold pellet weld to each other, the remaining channels of microporosity do not appear to be entirely confluent with one another.

Compaction technique for gold foil

Compaction begins when a piece of gold is placed in a tooth preparation. The gold is first pressed to place by hand; then a condenser of suitable size is used to begin malleting in the center of the mass. Each succeeding step of the condenser overlaps the previous one as the condenser is moved towards the periphery. The gold moves under the nib face of the condenser, effecting compaction as malleting proceeds.

The most efficient compaction occurs directly under nib face. Some compaction also occurs by lateral movement of the gold against surrounding preparation walls. The result of compaction is to remove most of the void space from within each increment of gold, to compact gold into line & point angles & against walls, & to attach it to any previously placed gold via cohesion.

The line of force is important when any gold is compacted. The line of force is that direction through which the force is delivered – the direction in which the condenser is aimed.

Compaction technique for E-Z Gold

Using an amalgam condenser or a gold foil condenser, the first pellet of E-Z Gold is pressed into the depth of tooth preparation & tamped into position.

A small condenser is then selected to thrust & wedge the gold into opposing line angles & against opposing walls to secure the mass in the preparation. Additional pellets are added,until the entire preparation is filled. To avoid creation of large void spaces in the restoration, a dense, fully condensed surface is obtained with each pellet before subsequent pellets are added.

Finishing of gold foil restoration

The first step in finishing procedure is to burnish the gold. A flat beavertail burnisher is used with heavy hand pressure to harden the surface gold. A cleoid-discoid carver is used to continue the burnishing process & remove excess gold on the cavo-surface margin. The cleoid, always directed so that a portion of the working edge is over or resting on enamel adjacent to or near the margins, is pulled from gold to tooth across the surface. This is done to smooth the surface and trim away excess gold. If considerable excess gold has been compacted, a green stone may be necessary to remove excess in class I restorations.

After the cleoid-discoid, a small round finishing bur (no. 9004) is used to begin polishing. It is followed by application of flour of pumice & tin oxide or white rouge. These powdered abrasives are applied dry, with a webless, soft rubber cup in a low handpiece. Light pressure to be used. Gentle blasts of air cool the surface during polishing.

NOTES

Section–2

ENDODONTICS

11 Clinical Diagnosis Methods

L.Q.A.1 Discuss in detail the various diagnostic methods used in endodontics?

Ans. The various diagnostic methods used in endodontics are:

PATIENT'S HISTORY

Subjective Symptoms

These are those which patient tell the dentist and includes pain / swelling etc.

Pain: The most common complaint that leads to dental treatment is pains.

It should be described under following parameters like type, onset, duration, aggravating, relieving factors, intensity (mild / moderate, severe), location.

Type I	Sharp Throbbing	Dentinal pain through 'c' fibers.
Duration	Transient	Reversible pulpitis.
	Continuous	Irreversible pulpal damage.
	Spantaneous (Without any irritating stimulus.)	Irreversible pulpitis.

CLINICAL EXAMINATION

Objective Symptoms

These are determined by tests and observations performedby the clinician.

These tests are:

- Visual and tactile inspection.
- Percussion.
- Palpation.
- Mobility and depressibility.
- Radiograph.
- Electric pulp test.
- Thermal tests (heat and cold)
- Anesthetic test.
- Test cavity.

Visual and tactile Inspection

One should do a through visual and tactile examination of hard and soft tissues and stress the importance on 3C^s i.e. colour, contour & consistency. Tooth should be inspected for its dullness, translucency, contour, fractures, wear facets and restorations. All this requires clean and dry field, good sight, good illumination. Instruments used are mouth mirror, probe, explorer, periodontal probe. Another important thing is to look whether the tooth is restorable or non-restorable.

Percussion

- It enables one to evaluate the status of periodontium surrounding a tooth.
- The tooth should be tapped lightly with the handle of the instrument.
- If the tooth is tender, it can be seen by patient's response in the form of blinking of eyes.
- A +ve response indicates presence of periodontitis (apical).

Palpation

It is done with fingertip using light pressure to examine:

- Tissue consistency.
- Pain response,
- Extent of swelling,
- The presence & location of adenopathy.

Mobility

Depreribility test - It can be done by the handles of the two instruments.

Grade I	-	Noticeable movement.
Grade II	-	Within 1 mm.
Grade III	-	Greater than 1mm.
		buccolingual + apical.

> **Note:** Percussion, palpation, mobility and depressibility are tests of the periodontium rather than of the pulp.

Radiographs

Radiograph is one of the most important clinical tool in making a diagnosis.

Limitations of Radiographs

- It cannot be used reliably to differentiale a chronic abscess, a granuloma or a cyst.
- Two dimensional image of 3-D object.
- Different opinions for interpretations by different people.
- Artifacts, superimposition of other structures.
- It cannot assess the exact size of the lesion.

Role of Radiographs

- They contains information on the presence of caries.
- They may show the no, course, shape, length and width of root canals.
- They show the presence of calcified material in the pulp chamber or root canal.
- Internal and external resorption can be seen on radiographs.
- Calcification or obliteration of the pulp cavity can be seen.
- Thickening of periodontal ligament, resorption of cementum and nature and extent of periapical and alveolar bone destruction can be arrested.
- They provide pertinent information concerning diagnosis, prognosis, case selection, instrumentation, obturation and repair of bone and cementum.

- It alert the clinician to impending difficulties caused by calcifications, periodontal problems, perforations, blockages and fractures.

VITALITY TESTS

Electric Pulp Test

Pulp vitality depends on blood supply but this test is based on stimulation of nerve.

The objective is to stimulate a pulpal response by subjecting the tooth to anincreasing degree of electric current.

Technique

- Isolation of tooth.
- Application of electrolyte (generally tooth paste).
- Application of electrodes to the tooth in question.
- First to the incisobuccal portion - If no response then to the middle portion and then to cervical portion. This is to provide minimal stimulus to the pulp and avoid injury.
- Testing of control teeth i.e. adjacent and contra-lateral tooth.
- Current is gradually increase with the help of rheostat till the required response is obtained and then stopped.
- Electrodes should not come in contact with gingival.
  - Interpretations sulcus, restorations, base etc.
  - Vital, Warmth, Tingling sensation, degree of pain, depends on severity.
  - Necrotic pulp, No response.

A positive response indicates that tooth is vital. It cannot tell whether it is normal or abnormal.

False Positive Response

- Moist gangrenous pulp.
- In multirooted teeth in which the pulp is partially neerotic with some nerve fibers still vital in one or more of the root canals.

False Negative Results

- Excessive calcification in the pulp tissue or selcrosis of dentin.

- Tooth with extensive restorations and a pulp protecting base.
- Recently traumatized teeth.
- Recently erupted teeth with incomplete root formation.
- Sedative medication taken by patient.
- Patient with unusually high pain threshold.

Thermal Tests

Heat testing and cold testing. Thermal tests are more reliable than any other tests.

A reaction or response to cold test indicates a vital pulp regardless of whether that pulp is normal or abnormal.

In short, +ve cold test → Vital pulp (normal / abnormal).

An abnormal response to heat test. Presence of pulpal or periapical disorder requiring endodontic treatment.

Technique

- Preparation of the patient.
- Invitation of tooth and should be dried.

Heat Test

- Generally hot gutta percha is used and applied to occluso-buccal third of the exposed crown.
- If no response then to central portion of the crown.
- If again no response then to cervical portion of the crown.

Note: Care should be taken to avoid using excessive heat or prolonged application of heat to the tooth.

- In case of hot water, tooth should be isolated under a rubber dam.

Cold Test

Methods:
- Stream of cold air.
- Ethyl chloride spray.
- Stiver of ice wrapped in wet gauze.
- Ice pencils.
- Dry ice.

Commonly ice is used as it is easily available.

Remember: Always control test should be performed on adjacent and opposite tooth.

Anesthetic tests

It is indicated when there is chance of multiple teeth involvement or when usual tests have failed to enable one to identify the correct tooth.

Technique

- Either infiltration or the intraligamentary injection is used.
- The most posterior tooth in the area suspected of being the cause of pain is injected first.
- Then the injection is proceeded forwardly one by one tooth.
- The process is continued until pain disappears.
- For differentiation of maxilla and mandible, an inferior alveolar injection should be given.

Test Cavity

It is performed when other methods of diagnosis have failed.

Technique

- A cavity is made by drilling through the enamel-dentin jn. of an unanesthetized tooth.
- With a round bur, slow speed, without a water coolant.
- If pain - tooth is vital. If no pain - tooth is nonvital.

S.Q.A.2 Enumerate the methods available for testing the vitality of a tooth ?

Ans. The methods available are:

- Electric Pulp Test.
- Thermal Test:
  - Heat test.
  - Cold test.
- Anesthetic test.
- Test cavity.

12

Endodontic Emergencies

S.Q.A.1 Explain hyperaemia of pulp

Ans. Signs and Symptoms -

- Sharp, Shooting pain usually by cold stimuli.
- Relieved on removing causative agent e.g. heat, cold.

Causes

Any irritant that can affect the pulp may cause reversible pulpitis or hyperacmia.

- Caries
- Periodontal scaling.
- Root Planing.
- Microleakage.
- Unbased restorations.

Tests

- Visual and tactile examination.
- Thermal tests.
- Radiographic examination.

Treatment

- Pulp protective base should be given.
- Marginal leakage should be avoided.

- All restorations should be contoured properly.
- Proper scaling
- Occlusal trauma should be reduced.
- Sedative dressings.

S.Q.A.2 Explain phoenix abscess

Ans. It is always preceded by chronic apical periodontitis.

Definition

It is an acute inflammatory reaction superimposed on an existing chronic lesion such as a cyst or granuloma.

Symptoms

- Tooth is tender to touch.
- Elevation of the tooth in the socket.
- Mucosa over the radicular area may be sensitive to palpation & may appear red and swollen.

Diagnosis

- Well defined periradicular lesion is seen radio-graphically.
- Vitality tests - Negative.
- Most commonly associated with the initiation of root canal therapy in a completely asymptomatic tooth.

Differential diagnosis - Acute alveolar abscess.

Treatment

- Drainage.
- Control of systemic reaction.

13 Diseases of The Dental Pulp

L.Q.A.1 Describe pulpal necrosis & their management ?

Ans.

Definition

Necrosis is death of the pulp. It may be partial or total.

Type

- Coagulation.
- Liquefaction.

Coagulation

In Coagulation necrosis, the soluble portion of tissue is precipitated or is converted into a cheesy mass consisting chiefly of coagulated proteins, fats and water.

Liquefaction

Liquefaction necrosis results when proteolytic enzymes convert the tissue into a softened mass, a liquid or amorphous debris.

Causes

Any noxious insult injurious to the pulp such as bacteria, trauma and chemical irritation.

Symptoms

- Discoloration of tooth.

- Non vital tooth.
- Sometimes H/O irreversible pulpitis.

Tests

- Thermal test.
- Electric pulp test
- Test cavity, (all are -ve)
- In partial necrosis thermal test +ve.

Treatment

Preparation and obturation of the root canals followed by bleaching of the tooth.

L.Q.A.2 Eneumerate the various causes of pulp diseases and Describe the clinical features and management of irreversible pulpitis

Ans. Causes

- Physical causes.
- Chemical causes.
- Bacterial causes.

Physical causes

Mechanical:

Trauma:

- Accidental (contact sports)
- Iatrogenic dental procedures (Wedging of teeth, cavity or crown preparation etc.
- Pathologic wear (attrition, abrasion etc.)
- Crack through body of tooth (Cracked tooth syndrome)
- Barometric changes (barodontalgia)

Thermal:

- Heat from cavity preparation at either low or high speed.
- Exothermic heat from the setting of cement.

- Conduction of heat and cold through deep fillings without a protective base.
- Frictional heat caused by polishing a restoration.
- ***Electrical:*** Galvanic current from dissimilar metallic fillings.

Chemical causes

- Phosphoric acid, acrylic monomer etc.
- Erosion (acids).

Bacterial causes

- Toxnis associated with caries.
- Direct invasion of pulp from caries or trauma.
- Microbrial colonization in the pulp by blood borne microorganisms (anachoresis).

IRREVERSIBLE PULPITIS

It is a persistent inflammatory condition of the pulp, symptomatic or asymptomatic caused by a noxious stimulus.

Clinical Features

- Paroxysm of pain by sudden temperature changes particularly cold, sweet or acid foodstuffs, pressure from packing food into a cavity or suction exerted by the tongue or check.
- The pain often continues when the cause has been removed.
- Pain is sharp, piercing or shooting and is severe.
- It may be intermittent or continuous.
- Pain exacerbates on lying down. In later stages, pain is more severe and is generally described as boring, growing or throbbing.
- Pain is increased by heat and is sometimes relieved by cold, although continued cold may intensify the pain.

Diagnosis

In early stages, thermal test are +ve. In later stages, thermal test are feebly reactive. Electric pulp test has abnormal response.

Treatment

- Complete removal of pulp or pulpectomy.
- Placement of intracanal medicament such as eugenol.
- In case of posterior teeth and there is shortage of time, pulpotomy followed by placement of a formocresol over radicular pulp.
- Obturation of root canals.

NOTES

14 Pulputomy and Apexification

L.Q.A.1 Define Pulpotomy. Give indications and procedures of the same in a permanent lower first molar.

Ans.

Definition

Pulpotomy is defined as the surgical removal of the coronal pulp.

Indications

- Pulpally involved children's permanent teeth in which the root apex is not completely formed.
- Childs posterior tooth with wide open apices that has a small, asymptomatic carious exposure.
- In child's anterior permanent tooth with a wide open apex that is fractured during sports or an automobile accident.

Techniques

- The tooth is anesthetized with local anesthetic. Before that other diagnostic tests should be done.
- Tooth is isolated.
- Access is gained.
- Roof of pulp chamber is removed.
- Bleeding is controlled with a moist pledget of sterile cotton.

- A long-shank spoon excavator is used to remove coronal portion of the pulp.
- The bulbous portion of the pulp contained in the pulp chamber down to the orifices of the root canals should be removed.
- The pulp tissue at the entrance to the root canals and that confined within the root canals should not be disturbed.
- The pulp chamber is next irrigated throughly with sterile water or with anesthetic solution.
- Pulp chamber is dried with sterile cotton.
- Haemorrhage is controlled with large, moist, sterile cotton pledgets left in contact with the pulp stump for 2 or 3 min.
- Calcium hydroxide is applied in the form of paste to the amputated pulp to a depth of 1 to 2 mm.
- Zinc phosphate or zinc oxide engenol base is applied over it.
- Then permanent restoration is done.
- Tooth should be checked with radiographs and vitality tests every 6 months.

S.Q.A.1 Apexification

Ans. Apexification is a method to induce development of the root apex of an immature, pulpless tooth by formation of osteocementum or other bone like tissue.

The rationale behind apexification is that the residual undamaged pulp tissue (if there) and the odontoblastic layer associated with the pulp tissue resume their matrix formation and subsequent calcification, guided by the reactivated sheath of Hertwig. Hard substance formed can be bone, dentin, osteodentin or cementum.

Technique

- The tooth is anesthetized and isolated with rubber dam and access is gained to the pulp chamber and root canal.
- Irrigation is done with sterile water or saline solution.

- Working length is determined using radiographs and should be atleast 2 mm short of the length of the tooth.
- Cleaning and shaping of the canal is done.
- After irrigation with sterile water, the root canal is dried with burnt absorbent points.
- Ca(OH) paste (thick consistency) is applied to the pulp chamber.
- With plugger, paste is forced into the root canal.
- The drug paste is forced into the root canal until the entire root canal is filled with $Ca(OH)_2$ paste.
- $Zn(PO_{21})$ base is condensed into the access cavity and composite restoration is done.
- Patient should be recalled every 3 months for radiography for calcific barrier.
- If no calcific barrier seen then fresh layer of $Ca(OH)_2$ is applied after the removal of old one.
- Root canal is obturated after completion of apexification.

NOTES

15 Rationale of Endodontic Treatment

L.Q.A.1 What is the rationale of endodontics? Give indication and contraindications of root canal treatment.

Ans. The rationale of endodontics is to remove the reservoir of bacteria or noxious products by cleaning and shaping of the root canal and obturate the canal with suitable material to allow the periradicular bone to undergo repair.

Injury to the calcified structure of teeth and to the supporting tissue by noxious stimuli may cause changes in the pulp and periradicular tissues.

Noxious stimuli can be physical, chemical or bacterial and can produce changes in the pulp and periradicular tissues that are either reversible or irreversible.

Mild to moderate noxious stimuli may produce sclerosis of dentin, formation of reparative dentin or reversible inflammation.

Irreversible inflammatory changes caused by severe injury can lead to necrosis of the pulp and subsequent pathologic changes in the periradicular tissues. Tissue changes following inflammation are either degenerative of proliferative.

Degenerative changes in the pulp may be fibrous, resorptive ir calcific or may give rise to suppuration.

Proliferative changes occurs when irritants are mild enough to act as stimulants and results in formation of fibrous tissue.

The reaction of periradicular tissues to noxious products of tissue necrosis, bacterial products and antigenic agents from the root canal has been desribed by Fish.

Fish had found 4 zones of reactions

- Zone of infections.
- Zone of contamination.
- Zone if irritation.
- Zone of stimulation.

The root canal is the seat of infection. The toxic products of microorganisms and neciosis pulps an irritating and destructive to the periradicular tissue. Therefore canal treatment is done to eliminate these force products.

Indications of root canal treatment

- Irreversible pulpitis due to caries.
- Traumatic injury to pulp.
- Non-vital tooth.
- Intentional due to prosthetic treatment.
- Internal resorption.

Contraindications

- Poor periodontal support.
- Non-restorable tooth.
- Obtruction due to dentinal sclerosis tortuous canal, pulp stone, broken instruments within the canal.
- Accidental or pathologic perforation of the root surface.
- Lack of skill.

16 Principles of Endodontic Treatment

L.Q.A.1 Discuss sterilization in endodontics ?

Ans. **Method** - The methods of sterilization in endodontics are:

- Steam under pressure.
- Chemical vapor under pressure.
- Dry heat.
- Glutaraldehyde solutions.

Steam under pressure

- E.g. is autoclave. It is the most common means of sterilization except when penetration of steam is limited or heat and moisture damage is a problem.
- The temperature kept is 121°C at 15 pounds pressure and the time required is 15 minutes.

Unsaturated chemical vapor under pressure

- This system is also called a Harvey chemiclave or chemical vapor sterilizer.
- The principle is that although some water is necessary to catalyze the destruction of all microorganisms in a relatively short period of time, water saturation is not necessary.
- It also kills microorganism by destroying vital protein systems like autoclave.

- It uses a solution containing specific amounts of various alcohols, acetone, ketone and formaldehyde and a water content well below the 15% level.
- The temperature is kept at 132°C at 20 psi pressure and time required is 20 minutes.
- Each time a fresh solution is required.

Advantages

- It will not corrode metals.
- Load comes out dry.

Dry Heat

It kills microorganisms primarily through an oxidation process.

Hot Salt Sterilizer

- It consists of a metal cup in which table salt is kept at a temperature between 425°F to 475°F.
- It sterilizes broaches, files and reamers in 5 sec and absorbent points and cotton pellets in 10 sec.
- It has an advantage over glass bead sterilizer in that glass beads clung occassionally to a net instrument and cause blockage of the canal.
    - Also the salt is readily available.
    - The salt used is commercial table salt and in addition contains a small amount of (1%) of sodium silicoaluminate magnesium carbonate or sodium carbonate, so it pours more readily and will not be fused under heat.
    - The salt should be changed weekly.
    - Instruments should be kept before atleast 1/4 inch below salt surface.

Glass Bead Sterilizer

- The mechanism is same as hot salt sterilizer except some differences. Instead of salt, glass beads less than 1 mm in diameters are used.
- Conductivity of heat in glass bead is less than hot salt sterilizer since air space are more.

Glutaraldehyde

- The instruments sensitive to heat is sterilized by this method.
- In takes 6-10 hrs. depending on the product used.
- For sterilization instruments remains submerged in glutaraldehyde.

S.Q.A.1 Describe components of rubber dam kit and advantages of rubber dam in endodontics ?

Ans. The components of rubber dam kit are:

Rubber Dam Material

Available in 5x5 inch or 6x6 inch sheets. Thickness of sheet are thin, medium, heavy, extraheavy amd special heavy.

Holder

It maintains the borders of the rubber dam in position.

Retainer

It consists of four prongs and two jaws connected by a bow. It is used to anchor the dam to the most posterior tooth to be isolated.

Punch

Used to punch holes in rubber dam sheet.

Retainer Forceps

It is used both for placement and removal of the retainer from the tooth.

NAPKIN

Lubricant

It facilitates the passing of the dam septa through the proximal contacts.

Modelling Compound

Sometimes used to secure the retainer to the tooth.

Anchors

It may be used other than retainers.

Advantages

Rubber Dam in Endodontics are:

- Patient is protected from aspiration or from swallowing of instruments, tooth debris, medicaments and irrigating solutions.
- Isolation of the working tooth.
- Soft tissues are retracted and protected.
- Visibility is improved. It provides a dry field and reduces mirror fogging.
- Efficiency is increased.

S.Q.A.2 Principles of endodontic treatment

Ans. There are 14 principles of endodontic treatment:

- An aseptic technique should be followed in all cases of root canal treatment.
- Instruments should be confined to root canal so as not to injure periapical tissue.
- A root canal should first be entered by a fine smooth canal instrument to minimize the possibility of forcing infected debris through the apical foramen.
- In practically all cases the root canal needs to be enlarged even though it may be fairly wide already.
- The root canal should be flooded with an antiseptic solution during instrumentation.
- The antimicrobial agent used for disinfecting the root canal should be non irritating to the periapical tissues.
- A fistula requires no special treatment.
- In all cases of root canal treatment a negative culture should be obtained.
- The method of filing a root canal is immaterial provided a permanently tight seal is obtained.
- The root canal filling should be acceptable to the periapical tissue.

- In the case of an acute alveolar abscess, drainage must be established for an adequate length of time.
- The incision should be made only when the swelling is soft and fluctuant.
- An injection into an infected area should not be made whether it be a LA alone or a combination of LA with an antibiotic.
- Not all pulpless teeth are amenable to treatment, not are all the patient candidates for endodontic service.

NOTES

NOTES

17

Preparation of Root Canal

L.Q.A.1 Mention the various instruments used for root canal preparation. Describe in detail the procedure of your choice to ensure through canal preparation.

Ans.

Instruments

The various instruments used or root canal preparation are:

Exploring: To locate the canal orifice and to determine or assist in obtaining patency of the root canal.

Debridement: To extirpate pulp and to remove debris and other foreign material. e.g. Barbed Broach.

Shaping: e.g. Reamers and files.

Obturating: e.g. Pluggers, spreaders, lentulo spirals.

Procedures for Choice

Step Back Technique: There are three stages and they are:

Establishing the apical stop and preparing the apical section of root canal system

After determination of working length, circumferential filing is done and apical portion is enlarged upto 40 nos. except central and canines which is enlarged upto 50 no.

Stepping Back

- Larger instruments are then used sequently and each larger instruments used is set 1 mm short of the previous instrument thus orming a stepped preparation within the canal.
- It is essential tht after each step is cut the original instrument used to prepare the canal to the full working length is reintroduced to maintain patency of the canal.

Completion of Preparation

The middle and coronal section of the canal can be prepared either by filing or by using Gates-Glidden burs.

- A size 2 or 3 Gates Glidden bur is used.
- Copious irrigation is essential.
- The ledges created along the length of the canal by the step back technique are small but must be removed by filing with the last instrument used at the full working length.

L.Q.A.2 Describe in detail biomechanical preparation and the recent advances.

Ans.

Objectives

The objectives of biomechanical preparation is -

- To debride and disinfect the root canal system.
- To contour the root canal walls and apical tip, for the purpose of sealing the root canal completely with a condensed, insert filling material.

Technique

Techniques of Biomechanical preparations are:

Conventional

- Here after determining the working length, the pulp tissue or its remnants are removed using reamers and files.
- The canal is enlarged to 3 to 4 times the original instrument inserted or until white dentinal shavings are coming out.

- The degree of enlargement depends to some extent on width of tooth.
- The canal of narrow tooth such as incisor cannot be enlarged as wide as lower cuspid.
- In all cases instrumentation should be done in sequential sizes to prevent ledge formation and irrigation should be done regularly.

Step Back Technique: (See L.Q.A. No. 1)

Step Down Technique

- The primary purpose of this technique is to minimize or elimnate the amount of necrotic debris that could be extended through the apical foramen during instrumentation.
- First, removal of coronal debris and flaring of the straight section of the canal to done using Gates-Glidden burs.
- It is followed by incremental removal of pulp tissue from the coronal and middle two-thirds of canal, then to the full working length using loose fitting straight files in large to smaller sequence.
- The full length of the canal is smoothed finally to remove the steps.

Double Flared Technique

- Combination of step back + crown down.
- The pulp chamber is irrigated with Na hypochloride and a size 15 or 20 files placed one-third of way into the canal and removed.
- Irrigation is done to washout the content of the canal.
- Size 80 file with stop inserted gently without pressure to the same length and canal is filed.
- This is followed by introduction of sequentially smaller size file to a 1 mm greater depth.
- This sequence is continued until the coronal and middle 2/3rd of canal are prepared and irrigated.
- Size 15 or 20 file is placed gently to full working length and true working length confirmed radiographically.

- The sequence of instruments is then continued down until the full working length of the canal is prepared.
- This is then followed by the step-back method.

Ultrasonic and sonic techniques of root canal preparation

Ultrasonic System:

- The ultrasonic handpiece has a component which allows a continuous flow of irrigant solution to pass along file and its oscillating tip.
- They rely on transverse oscillation of the file at appx. 25000 cycles

  Sonic Handpiece: Operate at 1500 to 6500 cycles / mm, The difference is that sonic system uses water as an irrigant and does not usually require diamond files for the flare of the preparation.

S.Q.A.1 What are the differences between a K-type reamer and H-type file? Describe the preparation of an anterior root canal with hand instrument after access cavity is prepared ?

Ans.

- Reamers are made by twisting lengths of wire which have a triangular or square cross-section. Traditionally it is made from triangular blank.
- The nos. of flutes in a reamer is less.
- The basic action is half -turn twist and pull action.
- H-type file are made by machining steel blanks of round cross section to produce elevated cutting edges.
- It is used in pull motion.

Cleaning & shaping of anterior root canal

- Gross debridement and working length is determined using 15 size reamer and file.
- Chamber is flooded with 5.2% solution of sodium hypochlorite.
- All isntruments are set to the established working length.

- No. 20 file is inserted to the desired length and engaged against the dentinal wall with lateral pressure and withdrawn.
- 5. Circumferential filing is done.
- The no. 20 reamer is inserted and again filing is done.
- Irrigation is done.
- Larger file is inserted followed by reamer.
- In between each successive instrumentation periodic recapitulation is done to maintain patency of the canal.
- When apical preparation is enlarged to the size of a No. 30 file or larger and the next subsequent size will not reach the working length the preparation of apical third is finished.
- To prepare the body of the canal, the largest file that did not attain the working length is inserted until it makes unforced contact with the walls of the canal and the walls are filed once.
- Irrigation is done.
- A H file one or two sizes larger than the previous file is used to finish the instrumentation of the coronal third of the root canal.

Instrumentation is finished when

- Clean dentinal shaving appear (White).
- The irrigant is turbid.
- Walls are smooth and clean.
- Preparation shows continuous taper in a apical direction.

S.Q.A.2 Mention the various irrigants used in canal preparation. Discuss the use of intraoral medication in effecting sterilisation of root canals.

Ans. The various irrigants used in canal preparation are

- A stream of hot water (140 to 175°F).
- Physiologic saline solution.
- 30% solution of urea.
- Urea peroxide solution in glycerin.

- A solution of chloramine.
- Na hypochlorite (5.2%)
- Na hypochlorite in conjunction with ethylene diamine tetraacetic acid (EDTA).

Most effective irrigant is 5.2% Na hypachlorite. It is a reducing agent. It will act as alubricant, solvent of pulp tissue, antiseptic and bleach. It also has significant antimicrobial properties.

S.Q.A.3 Describe standardisation and sterilisation of endodontic instruments ?

Ans.

Standardisation of Root Canal Instruments

- Instruments shall be numbered from 10 to 100, the numbers to advance by 5 units upto size 60, then by 10 units upto one 100 or above.
- Each number shall be representative of the diameter of the instrument in hundredths of a mm at the tip.

  for e.g. No. 10 is 10/100 or 0.1 mm at the tip. No. 25 is 0.25 mm at tip etc.
- The working blade (flutes) shall begins at the tip, designated as D_1 and shall extend exactly 16 mm up the shaft, terminating at designated sife D_2. i.e. $D_1 - D_2 = 16$ mm.
- The diameter of D_2 shall be 32/100 or 0.32 mm greater than D_1. i.e. $D_2 = D_1 + 0.32$.

  e.g. No. 20 instrument has D_1 as 20/100 or 0.20 mm. and D_2 as $D_1 + 0.32 = 0.20 + 0.32 = 0.52$.
- This sizing ensures a constant increase in taper of 0.02 mm/mm length for every instrument regardless of size.
- The tip angle of an instrument should be 75 +/- 150.
- Instrument handles have been color coded for carrier recognition as:

No.	Color Code.
6	Pink
8	Gray
10	Purple
15	White
20	Yellow
25	Red
30	Blue
35	Green
40	Black
45	White
50	Yellow
55	Red
60	Blue
70	Green
80	Black
150	White

- Instruments are available in lengths of 21, 25, 28 & 30 mm.

L.Q.A.3 Mention various methods to assess the length of root canals and describe any one of the methods. or Describe working length. How will you calculate the working length of a tooth ?

Ans.

Working Length

The working length in endodontics is the distance between the apical constriction and an external reference point.

Methods of obtainig the Working Length

1. Tactile.

2. Radiographic.
3. Electronic.

Tactile

- It is the oldest and most commonly used method. The expert clinician develops a keen tactile sense and can gain information from passing an instrument into the canal.
- There is a sudden increase in resistance as a small file approaches the apex possibly because:
  - The unresolved canal constricts first before exiting the root apex.
  - It frequently changes course in the last 2-3 mm.
- The patient response is an important factor to be kept in mind. If the instrument is passed beyond the apex it usually responds with pain.

Radiographic method

Ingle's Method: It is the most commonly used method and involves the following steps -

- Measures the root length on the pre-operative R/G.
- Subtract atleast 1 mm safety allowance for possible image distortion or magnification.
- Set the endodontic ruler at this tentative working length and adjust the stop.
- Place the instrument in the canal until stop is at the plane of reference.
- Expose and develop the radiograph.
- On the radiograph measure the difference between the end of instrument and that of the root. Add this amount to the original measured length of the instrument extended into the tooth.
- If the instrument has gone beyond the apex, subtract this difference.
- From the adjusted length, subtract 1 mm to confirm with apical termination of the root canal at cementodentinal function.

Weine's Correction: Franklyn Weine further made an improvement in this determination as follows:

- If radiographically there is no root / bone resorption then adjust by subtracting by 1 mm.
- If periradicular bone resorption is evident, shorten by 1.5 mm.
- If both root and bone resorption are apparent, shorten by 2 mm.

Grossman's Method: Preoperative radiographs, the knowledge of working lengths of each tooth and digital actile sense are used to estimate a tentative working length, he instrument is placed in the canal and a radiograph is aken knowing the actual length of the instrument and /G lengths of the tooth and the instrument, the actual length of the tooth is calculated as follows:

$$\text{Actual length of tooth} = \frac{\text{Actual length of instrument} \times \text{R/G length of tooth}}{\text{R/G length of instrument}}$$

(d) *Xeroradiography* -

(e) Radiovisiography -

Electronic method

Three types are:

1. Resistance type apex locator.
2. Impedance type.
3. Frequency dependent.

Resistance Type Apex Locator

One of the apex locator circuit is connected to the oral mucosa through a lip clip and other side to a file. When the file is placed in the root canal and advanced apically until its tip touches periodontal tissue at the apex, the electric circuit is complete. The resistance is now equal to the preset value.

This method requires an absolute dry canal with no contaminants, exudate,pulp debris or hemorrhagic fluid. The file should not contact any metallic restoration or carious portion.

Impedance Type

It operates on a different principle which considers the tooth a long hollow tube closed over at the end (apex).

The tooth also exhibits an upper electrical impedance across the walls of the root canal which is greater apically than coronally. This phenomenon is caused by the presence of transparent dentin which begins to form at 17 yrs. of age and continues to grow throughout the life.

At the constriction, there is an abrupt decrease in the impedance across the root canal wall which the apex locator can detect. The unit indicates this as the endposition of the root canal in an analogue motor dial.

This type of apex locator uses a handhold return electrode instead of a lip clip.

Frequency Type

The principle behind this type of electronic apex location is that there is a maximum ifference between electrode depending upon the requencies used.

It can be used in the presence of pus, pulpal tissue and fluid. This is its major advantage.

S.Q.A.4 Access cavity

Ans. A well designed access preparation is essential for a quality endodontic result. A poorly executed access will make the procedure more difficult, compromising the final result and consequently, the tooth's long-term survival.

The objective of an access preparation os to create a smooth, straight-line path to the canal system and ultimately, the apex.

This allows for complete irrigation and ease of shaping and obturation.

Ideal access results in straight entry into the canal orifices with the line angles forming a funnel that drops smoothly into the canal or canals.

Intimate knowledge of tooth anatomy is mandatory to visualizing where the preparation should be made.

A through investigation of the cervical outline, tooth angulation and restorations is mandatory.

S.Q.A.5 Endodontic files

Ans. The various files used in endodontics are:

- K-type.
- K-flex.
- Flexofile.
- Flex-R-file.
- Hedstroem file.
- S-file.

As their name implies, there instruments are used with a filing action. The instrument is placed towards the apex and when some binding is felt, withdrawn while at the same time scraping along the wall of the root canal. The action is known as rasping and there is little or no twisting of the instrument in the root canal.

Furthermore, the instrument can be used in a circumferential filing action whuch is a modification of rasping.

The instrument is withdrawn and reintroduced alternatively around the perimeter of the root canal to prepare the major portion of the root lying coronal to the apical one third. The instrument can also be used in a reaming action where necessary.

S.Q.A.6 Spiral root fillers

Ans.

- These instruments are normally made from fine wire twisted to form a tapered spiral attached to a bur shank.
- They are used to introduce sealer into the root canal, but as they are engine operated they are liable to become wedged against the canal wall and fracture.
- The Hawes-Neos type is the only one recommended by the author. It is manufactured from a rectangular blade of metal and thus less likely to fracture. There is little to recommend the use of spiral root canal fillers in modern endodontics.

S.Q.A.7 Importance of determining the working length of a tooth during root canal treatment.

Ans. The canal length is the distance from the apical exit of the root canal to the reference point on the crown of the tooth.

The exact working length of the canal must be determined to establish the apical extent of instrumentation and the ultimate level of the root canal filling. It is generally accepted that if instrumentation is confined to the root canal and subsequentroot filling terminated at the apical constriction, there is a better prognosis than in cases overfilled or filled flush to the apex. The working length must be verified accurately, therefore prior to any instrumentation in the apical third of the canal.

S.Q.A.8 Recapitulation

Ans. It is a term used during instrumentation of the body of the root canal and refers to a return to the last file used in the apical preparation to maintain the patency of the apical segment while one cleans and shapes the body of the root canal.

S.Q.A.9 Girouraticus

Ans. These are engine-driven instruments can be used for opening root canals however they should not be used for canal preparation except as a last resort. The giromatic handpiece activates a stainless steel barbed broach or reamer in the root canal through a 90° reciprocating are at a speed upto 1000 cycles / min. This instrument may pack the dentinal shavings in the canal.

When compared with hand instrumentation, the giromatic was found to be less effective for preparing root canals.

S.Q.A.10 Endosonics

Ans. It consists of a piezoelectric ceramic unit that generates ultrasonic waves, which activate a magnetostrictive stack handpiece.

The handpiece holds a K-file or a specially designed diamond file that, when activated, produces movements of the shaft of the file between 0.001 and 0.004 mm. at a frequency of 20000 to 25000/sec.

This oscillating movement produces the cutting action of the file and creates an ultrasonic wave of sodium-hypochlorite irrigant solution, which is delivered along the side of the file into the root canal.

It also produces cavitation that is, the growth and collapse of bubbles, with a resulting increae in the mechanical cleansing activity of the solution.

S.Q.A.11 EDTA

Ans. The chelating agent ethylene diaminotetracetic acid, commonly called EDTA, was introduced into endodontic practice by Nygard-Ostby. It functions by forming a calcium chelate solution with the calcium ion of dentin, the dentin thereby becomes more friable andeasier to instrument.

EDTA is relatively nontoxic and only slightly irritating in weak solutions. It forms highly stable, soluble, metal chelates in combination with heavy metals or alkaline earth ions.

It has distinct antimicrobial properties. It removes smear layer.

S.Q.A.12 R.C. Prep.

Ans. It is a viscous chelator, its principle ingredients are EDTA, urea peroxide and propylence glycol.

Glycol is the lubricant that coats instruments and facilitates their movement in open canals containing calcific material or in restricted canals that exhibit various degrees of calcifications.

RC Prep. can be obtained in a large. Preloaded syringe and an appropriate amount is then expressed into a small disposable syringe for single patient use.

It encourages the flotation of pulpal remnants and dentinal mud that reduces the probability of blocking the canal.

Using R C Prep. inconcert with NaOel causes a ascent release of oxygen that kills anaerobic bacteria.

S.Q.A.13 Pieso Reamers

Ans. It is a type of power-driven reamers. It has long, sharp flutes connected to a thick shaft. It cuts laterally and is primarily used for the preparation of post spare when gutta-percha has been removed from the obturated root canal. Although many clinicians use pieso reamers to remove the gutta-percha filling during post preparation, it is not advisable to do so and thereby to risk disturbing the apical seal, accidently removing all the gutta-percha, or perforating the root.

L.Q.A.14 Discuss perforations as one of the major causes in failure of endodontic treatment

Ans. Perforations represent pathologic or iatrogenic communications between the root canal space and the attachment apparabes.

The causes of perforations are:

- Resorptive defects.
- Caries.
- Iatrogenic events during or after endodontic treatment.

Regardless of the cause, a perforation is an invasion into the supporting structures that initially incites inflammation and loss of attachment, ultimately this may compromise the prognosis of the tooth.

Perforation at or below the crest of bone certainly pose a serious threat to an otherwise favorable endodontic prognosis. The interdisciplinary team must decide whether to extract or direct efforts towards nonsurgical retreatment, surgical correction or both. Iatrogenic not perforations are common. Root perforation by engine driven burs and reamers occurs infrequently during post preparation, whereas the more frequent perforation of the curved not apex, caused by failure to negotiate the canal curature during instrumentation is often unrecognized.

The apical perforation precludes access to the last 3 or 4 mm of the canal. Untreated or unfilled, this part of the apical canal remains a focus of infection, resulting in ongoing periapical disease.

The causes of pathologic not perforation are root decay, internal resorption and external resorption. The clinician must differenciate between internal and external resorption, including peroration, because treatment procedures and prognosis are specifically related to this diagnosis.

18 Disinfection of The Root Canal

L.Q.A.1 Mention the various methods used to sterilize the root canal during root canal treatment. Describe any one method in detail.

Ans. Disinfection of root canal can be done by following methods:

- Cleaning and shaping.
- Chemical irrigation.
- Intra canal medicaments.

This is done to control the growth of micro organisms such as Gram +ve, Streptococci, Gram –ve, Organisms, Yeasts etc.

Intra canal medicaments

They may be grouped as:

Essential oils: eugenol.

Phenolic compounds:

- Phenol.
- Para-chlorophenol.
- Camphorated para chlorophenol (CMCP).
- Formocresol.
- Cresatin.
- Calcium hydroxide.
- N_2.

Halogens:

- Na hypochlorite.
- Iodides.
- Quarfernary ammonium compounds.

Frequency of Medication

Intracanal medicaments should preferably be renewed in a week and not longer than 2 weeks because dressings become diluted by periapical exudate and are decomposed by interaction wit the microorganisms.

Techniques

- Isolation of tooth with rubber down.
- Access cavity is prepared and
- BMP is done.
- Canal is dried and intracanal medicament is applied with cotton pellet dipped in it.
- Temporary restoration is given.
- It should be changed before 2 weeks.

19 Microbiology

L.Q.A.1 Describe in detail the technique of culture examination and its importance in endodontic treatment.

Ans. Technique

Taking the Culture

- The dressing is removed from the root canal and is discarded.
- Any residual antibiotic or antiseptic from the surface of the root canal is wiped with a sterile absorbent patient 2-3 times.
- A fresh sterile absorbend point is inserted in the root canal for a minute so that tip of the point will be moist when removed.
- The absorbent point should be removed by sterilized cotton pliers.
- Unscrewed the cap of culture tube and lip of the tube is flamed.
- The absorbent patient is dropped into the culture tube and cap is replaced.

For Anaeobic Culturing

- A sterile needle of a Luer Lok syringe is inserted into periradicular space and aspirated fluid is immediately inserted into a vaccum vial and transported for anaerobic culture. This is for peiradicular tissues.
- For root canal, an access cavity is prepared aseptically into the pulp chamber and a few drops of prereduced, anaerotically sterilized medium is injected into the chamber and pumped into

the canal with a sterile endodontic file and aspirate similarly as for periradicular tissues.

Culture

The various culture media used are:

- Brain heart infusion broth with 0.1% agar.
- Trypticase soy broth with 0.1% agar (TSA).
- Thioglycollate.
- Glucose oscites broth.

Transport medium

Transport medium used are -

- Viability medium for growth (VMG).
- Stuart's transport medium.

Importance

The importance of taking culture examination in endodontics are -

- It is the best indicator of whether nos. of micro-organisms are reduced during treatment.
- It monitors the effectiveness of the biomechanical and chemomechanical preparation of the root canals.
- It determines the effectiveness of the inter appointment medication and seal.

20

Obturation of Root Canal

L.Q.A.1 Write in details about obturation techniques of root canal treatment including the latest methods.

Ans. The objective of obturating the root canal is the substitution of an inert filling in the space previously occupied by the pulp tissue, to prevent recurrent infection by way of the circulation (anachoresis) or through a break in the integrity of the crown of the tooth.

Techniques

The various techniques of the obturation are:

- Lateral condensation.
- Vertical condensation (warm gutta percha).
- Sectional condensation.
- Compaction (MC spadden technique).
- Thermoplasticised gutta-percha technique.
- Chemically plasticized gutta-percha (chloropercha, encapercha) technique.

Lateral condensation method:

- It is the most common technique of obturating the root canal.
- A primary cone is inserted into the root canal to the established working length and it should fit snugly and should resist removal (tug-back).

- A radiograph is taken to recify the fitting of the primary cone.
- Once the primary cone is selected the canal is dried and coated with thin layer of cement or sealer.
- The apical half of the primary cone is coated with cement and is carefully replaced in the canal.
- A spreader is inserted alongside the primary cone and is pressed apically.
- An accessory cone is inserted in the space previously occupied by the spreader.
- The procedure is repeated till the canal is filled.
- Excess gutta percha is removed with hot instrument.
- Obturation should be limited to this coronal 1/3rd of the tooth.

Vertical condensation method

It is used with step back technique of root canal preparation.

Steps

- Master cone is selected and canal wall and cone are coated with cement and cone is inserted into the canal.
- The coronal end of the cone is cut off with a hot instrument.
- A root canal plugger is heated to redness and is immediately forced into the coronal third of the gutta percha.
- Some GP comes out. A vertical condenser of suitable size is used to condense heated gutta percha apically.
- The procedure is repeated till whole canal is filled.

Advantages

- Excellent seal of the canal apically and laterally.
- Larger lateral and accessory canals also gets obturated.

Disadvantages

- It takes lot of time.
- Risk of vertical not fracture is there.
- Overfilling of guttapercha beyond apex takes place.

Sectional condensation method

- This techniques uses a section of a gutta percha cone to fill a section of the root canal.
- A master cone is selected and is divided into 3-4 parts.
- A root canal plugger is heated and apical portion of GP is mounted on it and inserted into the canal coated with cement.
- Disengage the plugger.
- Filled in the same manner until canal is fully filled.
- If a post type crown is to be made, only the first or apical section is used to obturate the canal.

Advantage

- It seals the canal apically & laterally.

Disadvantage

- Time consuming.
- It is difficult to retrieve the overfilled section of gutta percha.
- Chances of voids between two sections of filled GP.

Compaction method: (MC spaddan)

It uses heat to lower GP viscosity and to increase its plasticity.

The heat is created by rotating a compacting instrument in a slow speed contra-angle handpiece at 8000-10000 rpm alongside gutta-percha cones inside the canal.

The reverse H file is used to compact softened gutta percha apically & laterally.

Advantages

- Ease of selection and insertion of guttapercha cones.
- Economy of time.
- Rapid filling of canals apically and laterally.

Disadvantages

- Inability to use the technique in narrow & curved canals.
- Frequent breakage of compactor blades.

- Frequent overfilling of the canal.
- Shrinkage of the cooled and set filling.

Chemically plasticised gutta-percha

Advantages

- This method uses chemical solvents such as Chloroform, eucalyptol or xylol to increase plasticity of GP.
- This highly plasticized GP can be forced into fine, tortuous canals where other solid-core fillings cannot be inserted satisfactorily.
- Most commonly Eucalyptol is used.
- The softened GP can be used to coat the canal wall with thin layer and same cone can be inserted and compacted.

Disadvantages

- Inability to control overfilling.
- Shrinkage of the filling after setting.

Thermoplasticized gutta-percha method

Advantages

- In utilises a electrically heated syringe barrel and needles ranging from 18 to 25 gauge.
- The plunger is designed to prevent backward flow of the gutta-percha.
- Thermoplasticised gutta-percha is heated from 70°C to 160°C depending on the method or material used.

Disadvantages

- Lack of precision in delivering the gutta percha near the apical foramen and not beyond it.
- Chances of voids if there.

The newer techniques utilizing thermplasticized gutta percha are:

- Obtura-II High Temp 160°C.
- Ultrafil.
- Thermofil / Densfil.

S.Q.A.1 Silver cones ?

Ans.

- It is used to fill fine and tortuous canals that cannot be filled properly with GP.
- They require the addition of root canal cement to compensate for their poor adaptation to the canal walls and poor sealing qualities.
- After primary silver cone is cemented accessory GP cones are condensed around it laterally.
- They are contraindicated in post type restorations.

Advantage

- Silver is stiffer and easier to insert into a fine, tortuous canal.

Disadvantages

- Poor lateral seal.
- Difficulty in retrieving the silver cone.
- Lower success rate.

NOTES

21

Bleaching of Discolored Teeth

L.Q.A.1 Describe the procedure of bleaching of non-vital endodontically treated tooth.

Ans.

Procedure

The procedure of bleaching of non-vital endodontically treated tooth are:

- Internal Bleaching
- Walking Bleach Technique

Internal bleaching

The tooth is examined clinically and radiographically.

- An intraoral photograph of the tooth to be bleached is taken with a corresponding tab from a ceramic shade guide placed next to it to record initial shade.
- The outline of the CEJ is determined by probing circumferentially.
- Isolation of tooth with one adjacent tooth with rubber down.
- The treatment tooth is ligated with dental floss at the gingiva.
- All obturating material, sealer, cement and necessary restorative material are removed from the access cavity and 2 to 3 mm of obturating material from the root canal also.
- The access cavity is irrigated with copious amount of water and dried well without dessicating.

- Resin modified glass ionomer cement is introduced into the canal and access cavity.
- The base is contoured to follow the outline of the COJ and it should be kept 1 mm incisal to it.
- It should be maximum 2 mm in thickness.
- A cotton pellet is placed against the internal labial aspect of the tooth
- Superoxol is introduced to the access cavity carefully with a syringe and a metal needle.
- The solution is heated with a bleaching wand at a low to medium setting or with a dry endosonic spreader. The temperature should be no higher than 15° F above body temperature.
- The procedure is repeated as required.
- The tooth is rinsed with coprious amounts of warer and a fresh dry cotton pellet is placed in the cavity and sealed with cavit.
- The patient is recalled after one week to assess the color after rehydration.
- The procedure is repeated if required.
- The patient is recalled in two weeks to place permanent, bonded composite resin restoration in the access cavity.

Walking Bleaching Technique

It is indicated when results of chairside internal bleaching have been inadequate:

- The steps in walking Bleach remains the same as in internal bleaching, the difference is that instead of superoxol we insert a mixture of sodium perborate and superoxol or sodium perborale and water.
- The paste is packed into the access cavity and sealed with a 2 mm thick layer of cavit to prevent intraoral leakage.
- The mixture should be left for one week or until the patient notices the tooth as light or slightly lighter than the adjacents teeth.
- The treatment may have to be repeated if necessary.